MCQs
for the
MFFP Part I

for the Membership Examination of the Faculty of
Family Planning and Reproductive Healthcare

Ali Kubba MFFP, FRCOG
Consultant in Community Gynaecology
West Lambeth Healthcare (NHS) Trust, London, and
*Honorary Senior Lecturer, UMDS Department of
Obstetrics and Gynaecology*

Helen Massil MRCOG, MFFP
Consultant in Family Planning and Reproductive Health Care
Optimum Health Services NHS Trust, London

E. Sheila Merchant MFFP
Consultant in Family Planning and Reproductive Health Care
Ayrshire and Arran Community Health Care NHS Trust, Scotland

Claire Smith MFFP
Consultant in Family Planning and Reproductive Health Care
Mid Anglia Community NHS Trust, and
General Practitioner, Thetford, Norfolk

Martyn Walling FRCGP, DRCOG, MFFP
General Practitioner
Boston, Lincolnshire

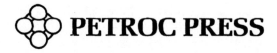 **PETROC PRESS**

Petroc Press, an imprint of Librapharm Limited

Distributors

Plymbridge Distributors Limited, Plymbridge House, Estover Road, Plymouth PL6 7PZ, UK

Published in the United Kingdom by Librapharm Limited, Gemini House, 162 Craven Road, Newbury, Berkshire RG14 5NR, UK

A catalogue record for this book is available from the British Library

ISBN 1 900603 00 4

Typeset by
Richard Powell Editorial and Production Services, Basingstoke, Hampshire
Printed and bound in the United Kingdom by
TJI Digital, Padstow, Cornwall

MCQs for the MFFP Part I

Contents

Preface

The stimulus for this book was the introduction of the new Membership Examination for the Faculty of Family Planning and Reproductive Healthcare of the Royal College of Obstetricians and Gynaecologists. The MFFP examination consists of three sections: Part I is multiple-choice questions and Part II consists of a modified essay paper, an OSCI and a critical reading paper. A dissertation will be required prior to sitting Part II.

This book concentrates on Part I, the multiple-choice question section. We have tried to follow the syllabus as much as possible, giving roughly the weighting of questions that we think the syllabus suggests.

So that the book will be valuable for general educational purposes as well as revision for the examination, we have included, wherever possible, extended answers to the questions. We hope that a wide range of healthcare professionals interested in family planning and reproductive healthcare will find this book useful in improving their knowledge of these subjects.

Finally, although every attempt has been made to ensure that the questions and answers are accurate, we accept all responsibility for any errors and omissions. We would be very pleased to hear from any readers who have any suggestions to improve the book.

A.K.
H.M.
E.S.M.
C.S.
M.W.

Acknowledgements

We would like to thank the following colleagues who contributed questions and advice on specialist topics: Mr Jonathan Aldis, Dr T. Biedrzycki, Dr David Boag, Dr P. Chowienczyk, Dr Gordon Downie, Dr Robert Hardie, Dr Helen Hutchinson, Prof Kenneth Norrie, Dr Elizabeth Ann Sankey, Dr Graham Sharp and Dr Giles Smith.

Section A – Applied Sciences

1. ANATOMY

A1 The cervix:

1. is relatively insensitive to cutting and burning
2. the uterine artery reaches the cervix via the uterosacral ligaments
3. pain from the lower cervix is carried via the pelvic splanchnic nerves
4. women exposed *in utero* to diethylstilboestrol (DES) show a cervical "hood" and a wide transformation zone
5. reserve cell hyperplasia is a consequence of combined pill use

A2 The following are components of the spermatic cord:

1. the cremasteric fascia
2. the testicular artery
3. the ilioinguinal nerve
4. the pampiniform plexus
5. the scrotal fascia

A3 The urinary bladder:

1. is extraperitoneal
2. the active muscle of the bladder is in the fundal part
3. has to be emptied before ultrasound examination of the pelvis is possible
4. is lined by epithelium sensitive to oestrogen
5. is closer to the urethral opening in women than in men

A4 The vulva:

1. lymphatic drainage is to the inguinal and then the obturator lymph nodes
2. the vestibule is the only mucosal component of the vulva
3. the vulva develops anteriorly from the cloaca
4. intraepithelial neoplasia is common from the vulval squamo-columnar junction
5. Bartholin's glands are usually palpable in the healthy state

2. HISTOLOGY

A5 Histology of the endometrium in the normal menstrual cycle:

1. the proliferative phase is characterised by prominent spiral arterioles and subnuclear vacuolation in epithelial cells
2. numerous subnuclear vacuoles signify that ovulation has taken place
3. menstruation is followed by regeneration
4. in the secretory phase there are dilated glandular lumens and stromal oedema
5. changes consistent with ovulation can be detected in 24 hours

A6 Histologically in the transformation zone of the cervix:

1. squamous epithelium of the ectocervix is replaced by transitional epithelium of the endocervix
2. in older and postmenopausal women the transformation zone is virtually always located above the external os
3. transitional epithelium is replaced by mucin-secreting columnar epithelium
4. there is a border between the stratified squamous epithelium and the mucin-secreting columnar epithelium of the endocervix
5. during the childbearing years and pregnancy the transformation zone is located in the endocervical canal

A7   In normal breast histology:

1. secretory changes indicate lactating breasts
2. normal acini are surrounded by basement membrane
3. myoepithelial cells found around breast acini are associated with inflammation
4. the epithelium lining acini (lobules) and ducts are histologically identical
5. the phase of the menstrual cycle can be easily determined by changes in the glandular tissue of the breast

A8   The normal prostate gland:

1. is divided into three lobes by well-defined fibrous septa
2. is composed of skeletal muscle and glands
3. has ciliated glandular epithelium
4. is devoid of nerves
5. is poorly vascular

3. EMBRYOLOGY

A9   Following fertilisation:

1. the zygote cleaves within 24–36 hours
2. the blastocyst implants into the uterus on the 4th day
3. the trophoblast invades the decidua so that maternal and fetal blood mix together
4. the fetal heart begins to pulsate during the 4th week
5. differentiation of the internal genitalia begins during the 6th week

A10 In human development:

1. the secondary oocyte has 23 paired chromosomes
2. at 12 weeks' gestation the fetus is 3 cm long
3. the transitional landmark from embryo to fetus occurs at 7 weeks' gestation
4. α-Fetoprotein is located in the fetal liver
5. differentiation of the external genitalia starts at 16 weeks

3

A11 Neural tube defects (NTDs):

1. are more common in Orientals and blacks
2. the incidence in England and Wales is 1 in 10 000 births
3. in most cases there is a family history of NTDs
4. the neural tube normally closes at 14 weeks' gestation
5. when a couple have an affected child the chances of recurrence are 20%

4. GENETICS

A12 The following diseases are autosomal recessive:

1. haemophilia
2. cystic fibrosis
3. achondroplasia
4. sickle cell anaemia
5. Tay–Sachs disease

A13 In Down's syndrome:

1. an unbalanced 14/21 translocation accounts for 40% of cases
2. the risk of recurrence after a spontaneous Down's-affected pregnancy is 1 in 100
3. the majority of babies with Down's syndrome are born to mothers over 35 years of age
4. the occurrence is 1 in 600–700 live births
5. the "triple test" is a definitive diagnosis for Down's syndrome

A14 In giving preconceptual advice:

1. the supplementation dose of folic acid to prevent first occurrence of neural tube defects (NTDs) is 400 mcg/day
2. chest radiography should not be carried out in the last week of the menstrual cycle
3. exposure to a noxious agent immediately after fertilisation can cause a congenital malformation of the brain
4. epileptic women should have folate supplementation throughout pregnancy
5. chronic villus sampling (CVS) leads to a miscarriage in 2% of cases

A15 Preconception counselling for patients with chronic schizophrenia should include:

1. a coital history
2. advice to avoid phenothiazines as they have a serious teratogenic potential
3. advice to commence a dietary supplement of folic acid 0.4 mg daily before conception and throughout pregnancy
4. encouragement to review their recent mental health with their general practitioner or local mental health team
5. the present evidence which suggests that there may be some genetic predisposition to schizophrenia

5. BIOCHEMISTRY

A16 The following ions are predominantly extracellular:

1. sodium
2. chloride
3. magnesium
4. phosphate
5. potassium

A17 Raised levels of serum prolactin may be the result of:

1. stress
2. hypothyroidism
3. Sheehan's syndrome
4. the use of oral contraceptives
5. chronic renal failure

A18 Recognised causes of hyperlipidaemia include:

1. alcohol abuse
2. hyperthyroidism
3. nephrotic syndrome
4. diabetes mellitus
5. pregnancy

A19 Which of the following statements regarding enzymes are true and which are false:

1. all enzymes are composed of one or more polypeptide chains
2. pancreatic amylase is important in the digestion of dietary protein
3. lactate dehydrogenase is present in human tissues in two isoenzyme forms
4. creatine kinase is present in both cardiac and skeletal muscle tissue
5. the activity of an allosteric enzyme is modulated by interactions between subunits of the enzyme

A20 Which of the following statements regarding vitamins are true and which are false:

1. vitamin B2 (riboflavin) deficiency is the cause of beriberi
2. vitamin B1 (thiamine) deficiency is one of the commonest vitamin deficiencies to be found in developed countries
3. vitamin C and vitamin E have antioxidant activity
4. vitamin B12 deficiency is usually caused by inadequate dietary intake
5. intestinal absorption of phosphate is impaired in vitamin D deficiency

6. PHYSIOLOGY

A21 Around puberty:

1. the prepubertal growth spurt is maximal in the year prior to the menarche
2. the rising level of oestrogen is responsible for the development of all the secondary sexual characteristics
3. the glycogen content of the vaginal cells increases
4. the action of lactobacilli on the glycogen of the exfoliated cells causes the vaginal pH to rise
5. the menarche is the beginning of regular ovulation

A22 In the normal menstrual cycle:

1. the proliferative phase is a constant 14 days
2. during the proliferative phase, the endometrium increases in thickness from 1 mm to 3 mm
3. menstrual blood loss averages 100 ml per cycle
4. just before ovulation, endometrial glands become tortuous and secretory
5. during the secretory phase, the cells become large and clear, and are separated by tissue oedema

A23 Ovulation:

1. is under the control of hypothalamic hormones
2. a rising level of luteinising hormone (LH) causes ovarian follicles to mature
3. the corpus luteum is formed from the follicle which has released an ovum at ovulation
4. the cells of the corpus luteum produce rising quantities of oestrogen
5. the corpus luteum begins to degenerate unless implantation has occurred by day 5 after ovulation

A24 The following are essential for myocardial cell function:

1. angiotensin II
2. calcium
3. sodium
4. magnesium
5. potassium

A25 The posterior lobe of the human pituitary gland produces the following hormones:

1. luteinising hormone releasing hormone
2. oxytocin
3. thyroid stimulating hormone
4. prolactin
5. antidiuretic hormone

A26 Physiological changes in pregnancy include:

1. an increase in plasma volume greater than the increase in red cell mass
2. an increase in total plasma protein concentration
3. a normal free thyroxine index
4. a 30–40% increase in cardiac output by mid-term
5. an increase in gastric and bowel motility

7. PATHOLOGY

A27 Concerning carcinoma of the breast:

1. breast cancer arises in the terminal duct lobular unit
2. malignant tumour grading is very inaccurate, and prone to observer bias
3. patients with a grade I tumour have an 85% chance of 5-year survival
4. special type (classic lobular, tubular, cribriform, medullary, mucinous and papillary) tumours have a worse prognosis than no-special-type (NST) tumours
5. the decision to use radiotherapy following mastectomy is based on tumour size alone

A28 Endometrial malignancy:

1. may occur in premenopausal women
2. is commonly preceded by simple cystic hyperplasia
3. usually involves a field change in the entire endometrium
4. can be associated with tamoxifen therapy
5. is more common in obese or diabetic women

A29 Exfoliative cervical cytology:

1. is used only to screen for invasive disease of the cervix
2. is used primarily to examine cells from the transformation zone
3. will show the presence of human papillomavirus (HPV) in 100% of cases where cervical intraepithelial neoplasia (CIN) 3 is demonstrated
4. may show false-negative rates as high as 30%
5. is an easier test to perform on postmenopausal women

A30 The following statements about ovarian tumours are correct:

1. immature and undifferentiated neural tissue can be found in benign teratomas
2. 30–50% of serous papillary cystadenocarcinomas are bilateral
3. ascites can occur in association with benign ovarian tumours
4. dysgerminomas are more common in women over 30 years of age
5. granulosa–theca tumours may be associated with endometrial hyperplasia or malignancy

A31 With regard to cervical pathology:

1. inevitable progression of cervical intraepithelial neoplasia (CIN) I to II to III is well accepted
2. cytological assessment of a smear is based only on the cytoplasmic changes of exfoliated cells
3. the cause of "cervicitis" is usually apparent cytologically
4. the presence of squamous metaplasia indicates premalignancy
5. CIN refers to a grading system for dysplasia of the grandular epithelium

A32 With regard to testicular malignancy:

1. the majority of teratomas are benign
2. spermatocytic seminomas have a worse prognosis than classic seminomas
3. a previous history of sexually transmitted disease confers a higher risk of subsequent malignancy
4. there is a higher risk of teratoma, but not seminoma, in undescended testicles
5. unilateral cryptorchidism increases the risk of malignancy in the contralateral testicle

8. MICROBIOLOGY

A33 Heat-sensitive surgical equipment and materials may be sterilised by treatment with:

1. phenolic compounds
2. buffered glutaraldehyde fluid
3. ethylene oxide gas
4. ethanol
5. ionising radiation

A34 Human immunodeficiency virus (HIV) is reliably inactivated by:

1. autoclaving
2. hot air oven
3. chlorhexidine
4. glutaraldehyde
5. hypochlorites

A35 Pelvic inflammatory disease (PID):

1. barrier contraceptive methods decrease the risk of PID
2. *Actinomyces* organisms are common causes of PID
3. after a single episode of PID a woman's risk of ectopic pregnancy increases
4. many women with PID have minimal or no symptoms
5. PID caused by *Chlamydia trachomatis* can be reliably treated with three doses of erythromycin or tetracycline

A36 The following can be used for skin disinfection:

1. quaternary ammonium compounds
2. phenol
3. glutaraldehyde
4. alcoholic solution of chlorhexidine
5. povidone iodine solution

A37 The following viruses cause vesicular rashes:

1. Epstein–Barr
2. rubella
3. measles
4. herpes simplex
5. varicella–zoster

9. IMMUNOLOGY

A38 Cell-mediated response:

1. is dependent on antibody production
2. T cells recruit and activate monocytes and other T lymphocytes
3. T lymphocytes combine with cell surface antigens
4. is the quickest mechanism to respond in an immune challenge
5. is the usual means by which foreign grafts are rejected

A39 Immunoglobulins:

1. IgG is the most plentiful immunoglobulin in internal body fluids and is produced during the secondary immune response
2. IgA is the major immunoglobulin in external secretions
3. IgM is the key immunoglobulin in the primary response
4. a polyclonal immune response involves the production of immuno-globulins expressing both κ and λ light chains
5. immunoglobulin-producing plasma cells are derived from immature thymocytes

A40 Immunology:

1. pregnancy is associated with depression of cell-mediated immunity
2. the human immunodeficiency virus (HIV) infects T helper lymphocytes by binding to the CD4 molecule and then fusing with the lymphocyte
3. an epitope is that part of an immunological antigen that binds to major histocompatibility (MHC) type II molecules on antigen-presenting cells
4. during pregnancy antibody-mediated autoimmune diseases of the mother do not affect the fetus because of the placental barrier
5. allergy to house dust mite is normally against the faeces of the house dust mite rather than the mite itself

10. PHARMACOLOGY AND THERAPEUTICS

A41 Absorption of orally administered drugs:

1. occurs mainly through gastric mucosa
2. usually involves an active transport process
3. completely determines the bioavailability of a preparation
4. can be accelerated by drugs that promote gastric emptying
5. is influenced by the polarity of the drug

A42 In pregnancy the following are acceptable for the indications given:

1. hypertension: methyldopa
2. hypertension: captopril
3. anticoagulation close to term: warfarin
4. anticoagulation in the first trimester: heparin
5. urinary tract infection: amoxycillin

A43 Teratogenic effects:

1. usually occur in the second trimester
2. when demonstrated in animals, preclude use of a drug in pregnancy
3. have been excluded when a drug is included in the British National Formulary
4. of phenytoin include craniofacial abnormalities
5. of stilboestrol include urogenital abnormalities

A44 The following are prodrugs:

1. 3-ketodesogestrel
2. gestodene
3. ethynodiol diacetate
4. levonorgestrel
5. norgestimate

A45 The following drugs can reduce the contraceptive efficacy of the combined oral contraceptive (COC):

1. sodium valproate
2. co-trimoxazole
3. rifampicin
4. acyclovir
5. cyclosporin

11. EPIDEMIOLOGY

A46 In obstetrics:

1. the definition of maternal mortality includes deaths within 1 year of the termination of pregnancy if related to, or aggravated by, the pregnancy
2. in developed countries haemorrhage is the most common cause of maternal deaths
3. the standard perinatal mortality is the sum of all fetal deaths and deaths in the first month of life
4. parity of 4+ is a risk factor only for low birth weight
5. up to 40% of maternal deaths in less developed countries are due to unsafe abortions

A47 The Pearl Index:

1. is the most appropriate way of assessing contraceptive efficacy
2. is expressed as a rate per 100 woman-years
3. is calculated by dividing the number of accidental pregnancies by 100
4. does not apply to emergency contraception
5. rises every time a woman drops out of the cohort

A48 The following statements are correct:

1. a cohort study investigates a population without a specified disease and measures the development of new disease in exposed and non-exposed groups
2. a cohort study is useful for measuring rare diseases
3. the RCGP Oral Contraceptive Study is the biggest case–control study of its kind in the UK
4. period prevalence is the proportion of people who develop a disease for the first time, over a stated period of time
5. the sensitivity of a screening test is defined as the probability of a positive test in people with the disease

Answers to Section A

A1 1 – T
2 – F
3 – T
4 – T
5 – T

The uterine artery reaches the cervix at the base of the broad ligament (2).

A cervical "hood" and a wide transformation zone are part of the benign vaginocervical changes due to diethylstilboestrol (DES) (4).

Reserve cell hyperplasia is postulated as one of the ways in which the pill may "promote" the development of cervical intraepithelial neoplasia (CIN) (5).

A2 1 – T
2 – T
3 – T
4 – T
5 – F

A3 1 – T
2 – F
3 – F
4 – T
5 – T

The extraperitoneal position of the bladder allows suprapubic catheterisation (1).

The active muscle of the bladder is the detrusor, which is at the base of the bladder (2).

The wide use of transvaginal ultrasonography improves the quality of the results without the need for a full bladder (3).

The urethra is 4 cm long in women and 20 cm long in men (5).

A4 1 – F
      2 – T
      3 – T
      4 – F
      5 – F

The lymphatic drainage of the vulva is through the iliac glands (1).

Bartholin's glands are not normally palpable as they are of a small size comparable to the size of a pea (5).

A5 1 – F
      2 – T
      3 – T
      4 – T
      5 – F

Prominent spiral arterioles and subnuclear vacuolation are characteristic of the secretory phase (1).

Sporadic vacuoles appear in some of the glandular cells immediately before ovulation but are unreliable as definite signs of ovulation (2).

Regeneration occurs after normal menstruation, anovulatory cycles, ovulatory functional disturbances or curettage (3).

Dilated glandular lumens and stromal oedema are characteristic of the secretory phase (4).

The first day after ovulation is morphologically mute because it takes 36–48 hours before changes induced by the progesterone secretion can be detected with assurance under the light microscope (5).

Reference: Dallenbach-Hellweg G, Poulson H (1985). *Atlas of Endometrial Histopathology.* W.B. Saunders, London.

A6 1 – F
      2 – T
      3 – F
      4 – T
      5 – F

In normal circumstances the transformation zone contains the squamo-columnar junction of the cervix, which is the border between the stratified squamous epithelium and the mucin-secreting columnar epithelium of the endocervix (1).

During the childbearing years and pregnancy the transformation zone is located in almost all instances on the exposed portion of the cervix.

Consequently, the vast majority of cervical neoplasias can be removed for histological diagnosis by punch biopsy (5).

Reference: Kurman RJ (1987). *Blausteins's Pathology of the Female Genital Tract.* Springer-Verlag, Heidelberg.

A7 1 – F
      2 – T
      3 – F
      4 – T
      5 – F

Secretory changes can be seen focally in the normal breast (1).

Myoepithelial cells are found around all normal acini (3).

Glandular tissue changes are a poor indicator of the phase of the menstrual cycle (5).

A8 1 – F
      2 – F
      3 – F
      4 – F
      5 – F

The prostate gland has no fibrous septa (1) and is composed of smooth muscle and glands (2).

The epithelium is cuboidal (3).

There are many nerves (4) and the prostate is very vascular (5).

A9 1 – T
      2 – F
      3 – F
      4 – T
      5 – T

The blastocyst does not implant into the uterus until the 7th day after fertilization (2).

The trophoblast invades the decidua forming villi. The maternal and fetal blood never come into direct contact (3).

A10 1 – F
      2 – F
      3 – T
      4 – T
      5 – F

The secondary oocyte has 23 single chromosomes (1).

A 12-week fetus is 6 cm long (2).

Differentiation of the external genitalia starts at 10 weeks (5).

A11 1 – F
    2 – F
    3 – F
    4 – F
    5 – F

Neural tube defects (NTDs) are more common in Caucasians (1).

The incidence in England is 1–2 per 1000 births and is higher in the north of England and in Wales (2).

Over 95% of NTDs occur in families without a relevant history, the cause being multifactorial (3).

The neural tube closes before 8 weeks' gestation (4).

The chances of recurrence with one affected child are only 5%. They rise to 20% after three affected children (5).

A12 1 – F
    2 – T
    3 – F
    4 – T
    5 – T

Haemophilia is an X-linked recessive disorder and therefore only affects male offspring (1).

The carrier rate for cystic fibrosis in the UK is 1 in 25 (2).

Achondroplasia is an autosomal dominant disorder. The risk of inheritance if one parent is affected is 50% (3).

The carrier rate for sickle cell trait can be as high as 1 in 4 in West Africans (4).

Tay–Sachs disease is a metabolic disorder that affects Ashkenazi Jews. The carrier rate is 1 in 30 (5).

If both parents are carriers of an autosomal recessive disorder, the risk of an affected pregnancy is 25%. Screening should preferably occur before conception, although at present all women are offered appropriate antenatal screening and their partners tested accordingly.

A13 1 – F
    2 – T

3 – F
4 – T
5 – F

95% of Down's syndrome cases result from a spontaneous trisomy 21, 4% from an unbalanced translocation and 1% from mosaicism (1).

Although greater maternal age is associated with an increased risk of Down's syndrome, 70% of affected pregnancies occur in women younger than 35 (3).

The "triple test", as with maternal age alone, gives only a risk for Down's syndrome (5).

A14 1 – T
2 – F
3 – F
4 – T
5 – T

Folic acid supplementation should continue to at least 8 weeks' gestation to prevent neural tube defects (1).

Chest radiography can be carried out provided the genitalia are shielded (2).

Exposure to a noxious agent after fertilisation has an all-or-nothing effect on the blastocyst (3).

Epileptic women are at higher risk of folate deficiency because of the interaction of antiepileptic drugs such as phenytoin with folate bioavailability. They should therefore have folic supplementation throughout pregnancy (4).

A15 1 – T
2 – F
3 – F
4 – T
5 – T

Chronic psychosis in one or both partners may be associated with sexual dysfunction, which may interfere with conception. Advice on coital frequency and effectiveness for conception can be offered to all clients (1).

There is no evidence that treatment with high doses of neuroleptic drugs throughout pregnancy is associated with a significant increase in congenital malformations. Some infants exhibit short-term neonatal toxicity but, as psychotic episodes during pregnancy are harmful to both mother and fetus, it is important that the mother continues to receive appropriate treatment with whatever drugs are necessary to control her symptoms. Phenothiazines may impair fertility if there is an induced hyperprolactinaemia (2).

The advice should be the same as for any other woman, i.e. folic acid supplementation is needed only up to the end of the first trimester of pregnancy (3).

Chronic schizophrenia can be a relapsing disorder and it is good practice to try to ensure that discussion about planning a pregnancy takes place when the patrient is relatively well. Patients who are receiving prophylactic medication may be advised to delay pregnancy until the mental state has been stable for a reasonable period of time (4).

Although present evidence suggests that there may be some genetic predisposition to schizophrenia this is compounded by family and social factors. If there is a strong family history of schizophrenia or if the partner is also schizophrenic, referral for specialist genetic counselling may be justified (5).

Reference: Watson C (1995). *British Journal of Family Planning* **20**, 117–120.

A16 1 – T
2 – T
3 – F
4 – F
5 – F

A17 1 – T
2 – T
3 – F
4 – T
5 – T

In hypothyroidism, increased secretion of thyrotrophin releasing hormone (TRH) increases plasma thyroid stimulating hormone (TSH) concentrations but may also increase prolactin secretion; this effect varies widely among individuals, but hypothyroidism should always be excluded in hyperprolactinaemia (2).

Sheehan's syndrome causes hypopituitarism, which results in normal or low prolactin levels (3).

The effect of oral contraceptives varies widely among individuals. Therapy may have to be discontinued to allow evaluation of the likely significance of the elevated prolactin level (4).

Raised serum prolactin is an almost universal finding in chronic renal failure (CRF). It may be secondary to the increased endorphin secretion found in CRF, but the link has yet to be definitely established (5).

A18 1 – T
     2 – F
     3 – T
     4 – T
     5 – T

Alcohol abuse is particularly associated with hypertriglyceridaemia (1).

Hyperthyroidism tends to cause lowering of cholesterol levels (2).

Nephrotic syndrome usually causes severe hypercholesterolaemia (3).

Particularly in non-insulin-dependent diabetes mellitus (NIDDM), which causes increased triglycerides with or without raised cholesterol. Younger patients occasionally have severe mixed hyperlipidaemia during episodes of diabetic ketoacidosis (DKA). This probably reflects a genetic predisposition to hyperlipidaemia in these individuals (4).

Pregnancy is associated with significant increases in plasma cholesterol. Most authorities would not recommend lipid-lowering therapy during pregnancy (5).

A19 1 – T
     2 – F
     3 – F
     4 – T
     5 – T

Amylase is important in the digestion of dietary carbohydrate. Enzymes involved in the digestion of protein include pepsin and trypsin (2).

Lactate dehydrogenase (LDH) is a tetrameric protein, each subunit existing in one of two forms, resulting in the existence of five different isoenzymes (3).

When an activator or inhibitor binds one subunit of the enzyme, a conformational change is induced which affects the activity of adjacent subunit(s) (5).

A20 1 – F
2 – T
3 – T
4 – F
5 – T

Vitamin B1 (thiamine) deficiency is the cause of beri-beri. It may also be associated with Wernicke–Korsakoff syndrome. B2 deficiency is associated with angular stomatitis, glossitis, pharyngitis and normo-chromic normocytic anaemia (1, 2).

This antioxidant activity may have a role in the prevention of ischaemic heart disease, a hypothesis which is currently being tested in clinical trials (3).

B12 deficiency is usually caused by failure of gut absorption of the vitamin, e.g. pernicious anaemia, Crohn's disease and coeliac disease (4).

Vitamin D has a role in the intestinal absorption of both calcium and phosphate; affected patients usually have hypocalcaemia and hypophos-phataemia (5).

A21 1 – F
2 – F
3 – T
4 – F
5 – F

The prepubertal growth spurt begins 3–4 years before the menarche. It is maximal in the first 2 years and slows down the year before the menarche (1).

The rising level of oestrogen is responsible for breast development, the deposition of fat in a female distribution, and growth of the genital tract (internal and external), but axillary and pubic hair growth are stimulated by androgens (2).

The action of lactobacilli causes a fall in the vaginal pH, leading to the acidic environment found in the mature premenopausal vagina (4).

The menarche is the onset of menstruation. This is rarely regular and often anovulatory in the early years (5).

A22 1 – F
2 – T
3 – F

4 – F
5 – T

The normal menstrual cycle ranges in length from 24 to 35 days. It is the secretory phase which is a constant 14 days, and therefore the proliferative phase is the phase of variable length (1).

Normal menstrual blood loss ranges from 10 ml to 80 ml, with an average loss of 50 ml (3).

The glands begin to become tortuous 2 days before ovulation but there is no secretory activity until after ovulation (4).

A23 1 – T
    2 – F
    3 – T
    4 – F
    5 – F

A rising level of follicle stimulating hormone (FSH) is required to mature ovarian follicles. The luteinising hormone (LH) surge causes ovulation (2).

The cells of the corpus luteum produce progesterone (4).

The corpus luteum degenerates if implantation has not occurred by day 7 after ovulation (5).

A24 1 – F
    2 – T
    3 – T
    4 – T
    5 – T

Angiotensin II is a peripheral substrate released by the kidneys. It has no effect on cardiac function (1).

All the others are necessary for myocardial cellular conduction (2–5).

A25 1 – F
    2 – T
    3 – F
    4 – F
    5 – T

Luteinising hormone releasing hormone (LHRH) is produced by the hypothalamus and stimulates the release of luteinising hormone (LH) and follicle stimulating hormone (FSH) from the anterior lobe of the pituitary

(1).

Thyroid stimulating hormone (TSH) and prolactin are produced in the anterior lobe of the pituitary (3, 4).

A26 1 – T
2 – F
3 – T
4 – T
5 – F

The plasma volume and red cell mass increase by 40% and 18%, respectively (1).

Owing to the resulting haemodilution the total plasma protein concentration falls; however, globulin concentrations rise (2).

Hence there is an increase in thyroid binding globulin levels, which offsets the rise in metabolic rate and thyroxine (3).

An increase in cardiac output is necessary to maintain the increased oxygen consumption (4).

Gastric and bowel motility are reduced secondary to the inhibitory effect of progesterone on smooth muscle (5).

A27 1 – T
2 – F
3 – T
4 – F
5 – F

The classification of breast carcinoma is constantly under review and has recently changed. Modern classification is according to histological features, but division into invasive ductal and invasive lobular types is unfortunate as it is clear that cancers arise in the terminal duct lobular unit rather than ductal carcinoma arising in ducts and lobular cancer arising in lobules. Carcinoma cells confined within the terminal duct lobular unit and adjacent ducts, but which have not yet invaded through the basement membrane, are known as carcinoma *in situ* (1).

Tumour grading by the Bloom and Richardson system has been standardised and is very reproducible. The grades are I–III and consider three components, which are each numerically scored out of three. These are tubular differentiation, nuclear pleomorphism and the number of mitotic figures present. The higher the score, the less well differentiated the tumour. Scores of 3, 4 and 5 are grade I, 6 and 7 grade II, and 8 and

9 grade III (2).

Grade I carcinomas of all types (no-specific-type (NST) or ductal) have 85% 5-year survival. Grade III NST or ductal carcinomas have only 45% 5-year survival (3).

Special type tumours have a better prognosis than NST tumours (4).

At one time radiotherapy was standard treatment after all mastectomies, but there is now a more selective policy, dependent on several indications:

- tumours larger than 4 cm
- high-grade tumours (Bloom and Richardson grade III)
- node-positive tumours
- node-negative tumours where there is widespread vascular or lymphatic invasion (5).

Reference: Dixon M, Sainsbury R (1993). *Handbook of Diseases of the Breast.* Churchill Livingstone, Edinburgh

A28 1 – T
    2 – F
    3 – F
    4 – T
    5 – T

Endometrial malignancy is preceded by atypical hyperplasia (nuclear and architectural) (2).

Malignant change is usually focal, often at the fundus, in an area of atypical hyperplasia, so that a scanty biopsy can miss a lesion (3).

Endometrial malignancy is commoner in obese women, as fat converts stored oestrogen metabolic products to oestradiol (5).

A29 1 – F
    2 – T
    3 – T
    4 – T
    5 – F

Cervical cytology is used to detect precancerous conditions of the cervix (1).

The transformation zone is an area of highly squamous metaplasia where cervical intraepithelial neoplasia (CIN) can develop (2).

Reference: Cuzick *et al.* (1994). Type specific HPV DNA in abnormal cells as a predictor of high grade CIN. *Br J Cancer* **69**, 167–171 (3).

Smears are often reported as negative but inflammatory. The presence of inflammation gives an unsatisfactory smear because the inflammatory cells may be so numerous as to make it impossible to see enough cells from the squamocolumnar junction to ensure that they are all normal (4).

The loss of oestrogen at the menopause causes the squamocolumnar junction to retreat into the endocervix, making it more difficult to sample adequately (5).

A30 1 – F
    2 – T
    3 – T
    4 – F
    5 – T

Immature and undifferentiated neural tissue is found in malignant teratomas (1).

Ascites can occur in benign fibromas (Meigs' syndrome) (3).

Dysgerminomas are more common in women under 30 (4).

Granulosa–theca tumours are hormone secreting (including oestrogen), thereby resulting in endometrial hyperplasia or malignancy (5).

A31 1 – F
    2 – F
    3 – F
    4 – F
    5 – F

Assessment is based on nuclear and cytoplasmic changes (2).

Often no cause of "cervicitis" can be seen (3).

Squamous metaplasia is a normal process in the transformation zone (4).

The system grades dysplasia of squamous cells (5).

A32 1 – F
    2 – F
    3 – F
    4 – F
    5 – T

Most teratomas are malignant (1).

There is a better prognosis in older age groups (2).

There is no relationship between sexually transmitted disease and malignancy (3).

60% of all malignancies are seminomas (4).

A33 1 – F
2 – T
3 – T
4 – F
5 – T

Phenolic compounds and ethanol are for disinfection only.

A34 1 – T
2 – T
3 – F
4 – T
5 – T

A35 1 – T
2 – F
3 – T
4 – T
5 – F

The most common cause of pelvic inflammatory disease (PID) is *Chlamydia trachomatis*. Treatment for this with erythromycin or tetracycline should last for 14 days.

A36 1 – F
2 – F
3 – F
4 – T
5 – T

Quaternary ammonium compounds have only weak antiseptic activity (1).

Phenol and glutaraldehyde are too toxic for use on skin (2, 3).

A37 1 – F
2 – F
3 – F
4 – T
5 – T

Epstein–Barr has the appearance of a pinkish macular/papular rash (1).

Rubella rash is macular/papular with occasional haemorrhagic elements (2).

Measles rash is slightly raised and macular/papular (3).

A38 1 – F
    2 – T
    3 – T
    4 – F
    5 – T

Antibody production is part of the humoral response (1).
The humoral response is faster (4).

A39 1 – T
    2 – T
    3 – T
    4 – T
    5 – F

Plasma cells are produced from B cells not immature thymocytes (5).

A40 1 – T
    2 – T
    3 – F
    4 – F
    5 – T

An epitope binds to immunoglobulin or T-cell receptor (TCR) (3).
IgG can be transferred across the placental barrier (4).

A41 1 – F
    2 – F
    3 – F
    4 – T
    5 – T

Drug absorption occurs mainly in the small intestines by passive diffusion (1).

Active transport processes are important for sugars, amino acids and vitamins and for a few drugs, e.g. L-dopa, methyldopa and lithium (2).

Bioavailability is the extent to which a drug enters the systemic circulation. This is determined not only by the degree to which the drug is absorbed but also by other factors such as metabolism in the liver before the drug reaches the systemic circulation (first pass metabolism) (3).

Drug absorption in the small intestine can be accelerated by drugs that promote gastric emptying, e.g. paracetamol and metaclopramide for migraine (4).

Lipid-soluble drugs are in general better absorbed (5).

A42 1 – T
2 – F
3 – F
4 – T
5 – T

Methyldopa has a well established safety record for essential hypertension in pregnancy (1).

Labetalol and other β-blockers are considered safe in pregnancy. Angiotensin converting enzymes must be avoided because they cause oligohydramnios (2).

Warfarin is teratogenic in the first trimester and may cause intracranial bleeding in the fetus following delivery if used close to term (3, 4).

A43 1 – F
2 – T
3 – F
4 – T
5 – T

The critical time for teratogenic effects is during organ development at 6–9 weeks' gestation (1).

Teratogenicity of new drugs in humans is usually unknown and for this reason they are not licensed for use in pregnancy, even though they are included in the BNF (2, 3).

A44 1 – F
2 – F
3 – T
4 – F
5 – F

Prodrugs are drugs that are converted to an active metabolite. 3-Keto-desogestrel is the active metabolite of desogestrel (1).

Gestodene and levonorgestrel are metabolically active progesterogens

(2, 4).

Ethynodiol diacetate is metabolised to norethisterone; norgestimate is metabolised to five major metabolites, including levonorgestrel (3, 5).

A45 1 – F
     2 – F
     3 – T
     4 – F
     5 – F

Sodium valproate is not a liver enzyme inducer and will therefore not affect plasma oestrogen levels. Most antiepileptic treatments are potent liver enzyme inducers, and therefore women taking these will need a 50 μg pill, possibly with a shortened pill-free interval (1).

Plasma concentrations of ethinyloestradiol are significantly higher in women using co-trimoxazole compared with controls.

Reference: Grimmer et al. (1983). Contraception 28, 53–59 (2).

Broad-spectrum antibiotics used in short courses will disturb the gut flora and affect the absorption of oestrogen from the bowel, making the combined oral contraceptive (COC) less effective. Rifampicin is a powerful liver enzyme inducer (3).

Acyclovir has no effect on gut flora and is not a liver enzyme inducer (4).

COCs will enhance cyclosporin levels, possibly raising them to toxic levels (5).

A46 1 – T
     2 – F
     3 – F
     4 – F
     5 – T

The definition of maternal mortality includes deaths due to abortion (1).

One of the commonest causes of maternal mortality is hypertensive disease of pregnancy, not haemorrhage (2).

The perinatal mortality includes deaths in the first week of life, plus fetal deaths (3).

Parity of 4+ is also a risk factor for antepartum haemorrhage (4).

A47 1 – F
2 – T
3 – F
4 – T
5 – F

In assessing contraceptive efficacy, the life table analysis is better (1). The Pearl Index is calculated by dividing the total accidental pregnancies by the total months of exposure multiplied by 1200 (3).

A48 1 – T
2 – F
3 – F
4 – F
5 – T

A cohort study is useful for testing multiple hypotheses simultaneously (1).

However, as the initial population is without the disease under investigation, a cohort study is not useful for detecting rare events. This is best investigated by a case–control study (2).

The RCGP study is a cohort study, not a case–control study (3).

A period prevalence is the proportion of people with the disease during a specified period of time. The definition given is for cumulative incidence (4).

Section B – Contraception

B1 For a healthy young couple using no contraception:

1. sperm survival in the female genital tract is rarely greater than 72 hours
2. conception is most likely when sexual intercourse takes place on the day of ovulation
3. successful fertilisation is unlikely more than 24 hours after ovulation
4. the average risk of pregnancy from mid-cycle intercourse is 50%
5. the pre-implantation wastage of fertilised ova is of the order of 30–40%

B2 The efficacy of the following methods rely mainly on ovulation suppression:

1. the combined oral contraceptive (COC) pill
2. the levonorgestrel intrauterine system
3. norethisterone enanthate injections
4. the progestogen-only pill
5. Norplant (Leiras, Turku, Finland)

B3 In advising about contraceptive efficacy:

1. in typical use, the condom and diaphragm are of equal efficacy
2. the efficacy of all contraceptives is age related
3. the lactational amenorrhoea method has a failure rate of 2–3%
4. the combined oral contraceptive pill has a failure rate of 0.2–8%
5. in ideal use, the progestogen-only pill is over 99% effective

B4   Regarding the acceptability of contraception in women with special needs:

1. an 18-year-old teenager with learning difficulty may be sterilised as long as consent is obtained from someone in loco parentis
2. Muslim women may not accept a method that prolongs their menstrual loss
3. Chinese women are less prone to thromboembolism
4. men with quadriplegia are unable to father children
5. recreational drugs reduce the bioavailability of contraceptive steroids by inducing liver enzymes

B5   In the immediate postpartum period:

1. sterilisation is associated with a high percentage of requests for reversal
2. the risk of venous thrombosis is higher than any such risk associated with the combined oral contraceptive pill in non-parturient women
3. both the combined and the progestogen-only pill can be started when the baby is 21 days old
4. the progestogen-only pill is ideal for lactating women
5. postpartum depression may be treated with natural progesterone

B6   With regard to women in their forties:

1. the overall maternal mortality rate is up to 10 times higher than that of women in their twenties
2. if the menstrual cycle is between 21 and 35 days the majority of women appear to ovulate
3. women over 45 years who have had amenorrhoea for over 12 months can consider themselves contraceptively safe
4. oral hormone replacement therapy has proven contraceptive efficacy
5. the combined oral contraceptive pill can control climacteric symptoms

B7 If a woman is HIV positive:

1. combined oral contraception (plus condoms) is a suitable method
2. an intrauterine device (IUD) is a suitable method
3. a female condom would reduce the risk of transmission
4. hormonal postcoital contraception can be given
5. injectables (Depo-Provera, Upjohn, Crawley, UK) are contraindicated

B8 In obese women:

1. the combined oral contraceptive (COC) is contraindicated when the body mass index (BMI) exceeds 40
2. there is a higher risk of failure of Norplant
3. menstrual irregularities are common
4. a high waist–hip ratio is an indicator of risk of cardiovascular disease
5. weight loss of more than 6 kg is of no consequence to barrier contraception users

B9 Older women:

1. having an intrauterine device (IUD) inserted at the age of 42 years may keep the same coil until the menopause
2. who are fit non-smokers must discontinue all oral contraceptives at 40 years of age
3. over 35 years of age who are smokers may take the progesterone-only pill
4. should have their IUDs removed 1 year after the menopause
5. depot medroxyprogesterone acetate (DPMA) is a suitable contraceptive for perimenopausal women

B10 In a woman taking phenytoin as an anticonvulsant:

1. an increased dose of the Yuzpe method is ineffective
2. should be prescribed depot medroxyprogesterone acetate every 6 weeks
3. could benefit from an injectable contraceptive if her epilepsy is exacerbated premenstrually
4. it may be necessary to increase the daily ethinyloestradiol dose to 100 µg
5. a higher-dose combined oral contraceptive pill should be continued for 8 weeks if the phenytoin treatment is discontinued

B11 Considering the cultural influences on contraceptive counselling:

1. Hindus prefer condoms to other contraceptives
2. Islam does not allow termination of pregnancy under any circumstances
3. male sterilisation is against the Sikh religion
4. diabetes is four times as common in Asians as in Caucasians
5. Rastafarians tend to follow the Old Testament teaching of "Be fruitful and multiply and replenish the earth"

B12 A doctor cannot give contraceptive treatment to a girl under 16 years of age:

1. unless she consents to him informing her parents or guardians
2. unless she understands the advice he gives
3. unless she allows a physical examination
4. unless she is already having sexual intercourse
5. in a family planning clinic without the consent of her general practitioner

B13 Menorrhagia:

1. is defined as menstrual blood loss > 80 ml per cycle
2. oral progestogen is the first-line treatment for ovulatory dysfunctional uterine bleeding
3. the levonorgestrel intrauterine system (IUS) reduces blood loss by over 80%
4. most cases are caused by hormonal imbalance
5. is a consequence of female sterilisation

B14 Combined oral contraceptives:

1. protection is reduced if the pill-free period is lengthened to 9 days
2. pills containing levonorgestrel should not be taken by women with varicose veins
3. should be discontinued at 35 years in smokers
4. may be given to women who suffer from focal migraine
5. there is no direct evidence that acute myocardial infarction occurs less frequently in third-generation pill users than in second-generation users

B15 Leiden mutation of coagulation factor V:

1. may be found in between 10 and 20% of patients with recurrent venous thrombosis
2. has been shown in recent research to be a *more* than additive risk factor when combined with combined oral contraceptive (COC) use
3. may be screened for with a clotting time test
4. causes activated protein S resistance
5. should be screened for in any patient intending to start using COCs if there is a family history of thromboembolism regardless of the age at which this thrombotic episode occurred

B16 The following are absolute contraindications to the combined pill:

1. herpes gestationis
2. previous deep vein thrombosis
3. moderate dyskaryosis on cytology
4. idiopathic jaundice of pregnancy
5. fibroadenosis of the breast

B17 The following are well-established non-contraceptive benefits of the combined pill:

1. reduction in pelvic inflammatory disease
2. improvement in eczematous skin disease
3. a 50% reduction in ovarian cancer
4. less peptic ulceration
5. 50% less benign breast disease

B18 Combined oral contraceptives (COCs):

1. women with severe acne can be prescribed gestodene- or desogestrel-containing COCs
2. third-generation progestogen COCs have been shown to have no effect on glucose tolerance
3. women using the same COC can show 10-fold differences in blood levels of ethinyloestradiol
4. diabetes is an absolute contraindication to COC use
5. high doses of ascorbic acid interfere with COC absorption

B19 Progestogen-only pills (POPs):

1. Microval (Wyeth, Maidenhead, UK) contains only one-fifth of the levonorgestrel that Ovranette (Wyeth) contains
2. antibiotics have no effect on progestogen blood levels
3. the older the woman the more contraceptively effective is the POP
4. Femulen (Gold Cross, High Wycombe, UK) contains the progestogen gestodene
5. the POP can be prescribed in women with recent trophoblastic disease even if the level of human chorionic gonadotrophin (hCG) is still raised

B20 Progestogen-only pills:

1. become effective within 48 hours of the first dose
2. are commonly associated with menstrual disturbance
3. are associated with functional ovarian cysts
4. are contraindicated during lactation
5. may give some relief from menopausal flushing

B21 Progestogen-only pills:

1. can cause erythema nodosum
2. can be prescribed to diabetics
3. in a breast-feeding woman, will reduce milk volume by an average of 10%
4. should be stopped before major surgery
5. offer some protection against pelvic inflammatory disease

B22 In advising about emergency contraception:

1. a copper intrauterine device (IUD) can be used up to day 19 of a regular 28-day cycle, even if three episodes of unprotected intercourse on days 6, 12 and 17 have taken place
2. following combined oestrogen/progesterone emergency contraception, 50% of patients would vomit at least one of the doses
3. the IUD is medically safer that emergency hormonal contraception for diabetic women
4. following emergency hormonal contraception, the start of the combined pill should be delayed to day 5 of the next cycle
5. the total dose of the Yuzpe regimen is equivalent to seven low-dose combined pills

B23 Emergency (postcoital) contraception:

1. is indicated if two combined contraceptive pills are missed mid-packet and intercourse occurs
2. the hormonal dose should be increased by 50% if a woman is on Amoxil (Bencard, Brentford, UK)
3. may be given twice in the same menstrual cycle
4. failure is an indication for medical termination
5. is not indicated if intercourse occurs 24 hours after missing a progestogen-only pill

B24 Injectable contraception:

1. is contraindicated in women with a history of ectopic pregnancy
2. is associated with functional ovarian cysts
3. usually produces endogenous oestradiol levels in the early follicular range
4. produces endometrial atrophy
5. reduces the incidence of pelvic inflammatory disease

B25 Depot medroxyprogesterone acetate (DMPA):

1. demonstrates first-order kinetics
2. is a 19-nortestosterone derivative
3. is formulated as microcrystals
4. can be given subcutaneously as well as intramuscularly
5. is more effective if the injection site is massaged

B26 The following are absolute contraindications to using depot medroxyprogesterone acetate:

1. severe obesity
2. lactation
3. phenytoin
4. active liver disease
5. systemic lupus erythematosus (SLE)

B27 With regard to depot medroxyprogesterone acetate (DPMA), the following statements are correct:

1. 50 mg intramuscularly every 12 weeks gives effective contraception
2. DMPA is licensed in the UK for long-term use "only in women in whom other contraceptives are contraindicated or have caused unacceptable side-effects or are otherwise unsatisfactory"
3. galactorrhoea may occur in women who are not breast feeding
4. enuresis may recur in women with a past history of enuresis
5. DMPA increases the risk of endometrial cancer

B28 Depot medroxyprogesterone acetate:

1. is associated with an increased haemoglobin concentration in long-term users
2. produces amenorrhoea in over 50% of users by the end of the first year
3. is more likely to produce irregular bleeding in women who experience such bleeding with the progestogen-only pill
4. may cause bleeding irregularities, which can be treated with conjugated oestrogens
5. may have long-lasting effects after the last injection: return to normal fertility may take 12 months or more

B29 Contraceptive vaginal rings:

1. are produced only in a progestogen-only formulation
2. of all types are worn continuously
3. have not revealed any surprising side-effects in trials
4. need to be fitted in the individual women in the same way that a diaphragm is fitted
5. the hormone carrier is made of silastic

B30 Norplant (Leiras, Turku, Finland):

1. amenorrhoea occurs in 50% of women in the first year
2. progestogen levels fluctuate on a daily basis
3. ovarian follicular development is suppressed
4. alopecia has been reported as a rare side-effect
5. difficulty in removal is directly related to the period of use

B31 Norplant:

1. consists of five subdermal silastic implants containing crystalline levonorgestrel
2. is highly likely to cause menstrual disturbance
3. has a contraceptive efficacy approaching that of female sterilisation
4. becomes cost effective at 2.5 years of use
5. removal takes longer than insertion

B32 Norplant:

1. can be used in women with endometriosis
2. contains 40 µg levonorgestrel per rod
3. is absolutely contraindicated if there is a history of an ectopic pregnancy
4. does not prevent ovulation in all women in the first year of use
5. may be associated with depression

B33 Women using an intrauterine device (IUD):

1. are at a higher risk of infection during the first year of use
2. should be advised to have it removed or replaced if *Actinomyces*-like organisms show on cervical smears
3. can have it removed at the time of sterilisation regardless of cycle phase or coital history
4. can be assured that all IUDs in current use are effective for at least 5 years
5. are at a higher risk of "inflammatory" changes in cervical smears

B34 The copper IUD:

1. should not be replaced in mid-cycle
2. causes ectopic pregnancy
3. is commonly displaced after a Pipelle endometrial biopsy
4. can perforate in 1 in 100 cases
5. has a failure rate of less than 1%

B35 The copper IUD:

1. should be removed in early pregnancy to reduce the risk of a later miscarriage
2. has a lower expulsion rate in nulliparous women than in parous women
3. increases the number of leucocytes in uterine and tubal fluid
4. may be used by a woman who has had subacute bacterial endocarditis
5. should be inserted during the fourth week of the menstrual cycle

B36 With regard to intrauterine devices (IUDs):

1. the risk of death is less with an IUD than with the combined oral contraceptive
2. if a pregnancy occurs, an IUD should be removed as early as possible
3. contraceptive protection starts 7 days after an IUD is fitted
4. leukaemia is a relative contraindication for IUD use
5. a copper IUD will be detected by airport security services

B37 Natural family planning:

1. pre-ejaculate secretions can contain sperm
2. sperm can survive *in vivo* for up to 6 days
3. at ovulation the cervical mucus is slippery and stretchable
4. following ovulation the ovum survives for 48 hours
5. the second infertile phase begins 5 days after ovulation pain

B38 Natural family planning:

1. the cervix is higher in the pelvis during the infertile phase
2. medication reducing nasal secretions reduces the amount of cervical mucus
3. with careful use the symptothermal method is up to 97% effective
4. a basal body temperature lowered by 0.2°C for 2 consecutive days predicts ovulation
5. the start of the fertile phase may be detected by monitoring the urinary oestrone 3-glucuronide

B39 Condoms:

1. Japan accounts for more than a quarter of all condom users in the world
2. double Dutch in contraception means pill plus condom
3. baby oil will not affect the strength of a condom
4. nystatin vaginal pessaries will affect the strength of a condom
5. the risk of developing cervical dyskaryosis decreases when a partner uses a condom

B40 Femidom (Chartex International, London, UK):

1. is a female condom made of polyurethane
2. should be introduced into the vagina immediately before intercourse
3. is spermicidally lubricated
4. has a high level of impermeability to virus particles
5. cannot be damaged by oil-based lubricants

B41 Caps and diaphragms:

1. the cervical cap stays *in situ* by suction
2. there is a reduction in the risk of developing cervical dyskaryosis in users of cervical diaphragms
3. Cyclogest (Cox, Barnstaple, UK) can damage rubber caps
4. caps should be left *in situ* for 12 hours after sexual intercourse
5. the Vimule cap (Lamberts, Luton, UK) is useful for long cervices

B42 Caps and diaphragms:

1. more frequent urinary tract infection is associated with the use of a cervical cap
2. Canesten cream (Baypharm, Newbury, UK) is not known to damage rubber caps
3. *Escherichia coli* is found more often in vaginal cultures of cap users than in matched non-cap users
4. occlusive caps can give effective protection against human immuno-deficiency virus (HIV) infection
5. a further application of spermicide is advised if intercourse takes place 3 hours after insertion of the cap with a spermicide

B43 Spermicides:

1. can be absorbed into the circulation
2. can be teratogenic
3. hyperkeratosis of the cervix or vagina can develop with spermicidal usage
4. spermicidal foaming tablets can be inserted just before intercourse
5. an 80 mg propranolol tablet inserted vaginally can act as a sperm-icide

B44 Vasectomy:

1. should not be performed on men under the age of 35 years
2. is not effective until approximately 20 ejaculations have cleared residual sperm from the semen
3. requires the consent of both partners
4. is associated with an increased risk of testicular cancer
5. is associated with increased libido

B45 In female laparoscopic "clip" sterilization:

1. the operation can be performed under local anaesthesia
2. the failure rate is approximately 2–3 per 1000 operations
3. there are no additional complications if the procedure is performed at the same time as a termination of pregnancy
4. an intrauterine device should be removed at the time of operation, even if sexual intercourse has occurred the previous day
5. a portion of each fallopian tube is excised and sent for histological examination

B46 The antiprogesterone RU-486 (mifepristone):

1. is licensed for terminating pregnancies up to 63 days' gestation
2. is used to induce abortion with a prostaglandin, which is administered 4 days after the RU-486
3. is used in a dose of 500 mg to achieve termination of pregnancy
4. has been shown by research to be effective for postcoital contra-ception
5. used alone will produce an abortion in up to 50% of women

B47 With regard to termination of pregnancy:

1. pregnancy cannot be legally terminated beyond 24 weeks
2. only one doctor's signature is required on the HSA1 form when the mother's life is at serious risk
3. the "all ages" legal abortion rate in England and Wales in 1993 was 12.3 per 1000 resident women
4. there is an association between first trimester surgical abortion and development of cervical incompetence
5. in pregnancies greater than 16 weeks' gestation, termination of pregnancy can be performed surgically or by means of prostaglandin pessaries

B48 A woman requesting a termination of pregnancy:

1. should have a cervical smear as part of the assessment
2. has a 30% chance of chlamydial infection
3. cannot have a medical termination if she is over 35 and smokes 20 cigarettes a day
4. should be advised of a 3% serious complication risk of suction termination of pregnancy
5. should be advised that failure to terminate a pregnancy occurs in 1–3 in 1000 cases

B49 Family planning practice and the law:

1. negligent provision of family planning services leads to no legally recognised loss
2. negligence in law is the failure to achieve the standard of the ordinary reasonable specialist
3. if a patient is sterilised without consent there is no legal wrong committed so long as the surgeon is acting in the best interests of the patient
4. family planning procedures can be provided to a married person even without the consent of the partner
5. postcoital birth control is legally abortion because it prevents the implantation of a fertilised egg rather than preventing fertilisation

Answers to Section B

B1 1 – F
     2 – F
     3 – T
     4 – F
     5 – T

In terms of fertility, it is the strongest sperms which are relevant. Survival is common for 5 days, and may occasionally be 7 days (1).

Studies have shown that the highest conception rate occurs when sexual intercourse takes place 2 days before ovulation (2).

Ova are fertilisable for only 12–24 hours after release from the ovary (3).

The average risk of pregnancy from mid-cycle exposure is 30% (4).

B2 1 – T
     2 – F
     3 – T
     4 – F
     5 – F

The efficacy of the levonorgestrel intrauterine system mainly relies on endometrial atrophy and thickening of the cervical mucus. Ovulation is suppressed in approximately 20% of cycles (2).

The efficacy of the progestogen-only pill and Norplant relies mainly on thickening of the cervical mucus (4, 5).

B3 1 – F
     2 – T
     3 – T
     4 – T
     5 – T

The failure rate of diaphragms can be up to 18% in typical use and is therefore higher than the failure rate for a condom (1).

All methods of contraception are more effective in older women (2).

B4 1 – F
    2 – T
    3 – T
    4 – F
    5 – F

The consent of a parent is not adequate to allow the sterilization of an "adult" with a learning difficulty. The level of mental competency of the individual, her prospects and her social wellbeing have to be considered, and expert views are routinely obtained (1).

Men with quadriplegia can father children with the help of assisted conception techniques (4).

A potential effect of recreational drugs on bioavailability of systemic contraceptives is through dehydration (5).

B5 1 – T
    2 – T
    3 – T
    4 – T
    5 – F

Regret after postpartum sterilisation can reach up to 5% *versus* 1% for interval sterilisation (1).

Postpartum depression may be treated with natural oestrogens (5).

B6 1 – T
    2 – T
    3 – T
    4 – F
    5 – T

Maternal mortality rate increases with age and parity. However, the age-specific mortality rates for primiparous mothers are higher than in a second pregnancy. (Spontaneous abortion and perinatal mortality rates are double those of women in their twenties.)

Reference: Report on Confidential Enquiries into Maternal Deaths in England and Wales. HMSO, London (1).

Increasing cycle lengths are associated with a diminishing incidence of ovulation. However, in women over 40 with regular cycles, 93% appear to ovulate, although pregnancy rates remain low due to an inadequate luteal phase (2).

Oral hormone replacement therapy (HRT) has not been consistently shown to suppress ovulation. Oestrogen implants (100 mg) with cyclical progesterone suppresses ovulation, although there may be a delay in action in some cases. HRT is not licensed for contraceptive use at the moment (4).

Reference: Bowen-Simpkins P (1991). Contraception for the older woman. In: Filshie M, Guillebaude J (eds) *Contraception – Science and Practice.* Butterworths, London.

B7   1 – T
    2 – F
    3 – T
    4 – T
    5 – F

It has been largely discounted that the combined oral contraceptive pill (COC) might facilitate human immunodeficiency virus (HIV) transmission. In fact, COCs reduce the risk of pelvic inflammatory disease and may therefore reduce the risk of HIV infection indirectly – as HIV infection risk increases when other sexually transmitted diseases are present (1).

There is an increased risk of severe infection (2).

A female condom provides a barrier for both the vagina and the vulva (3).

Effective postcoital contraception may be particularly important in HIV-positive women (4).

Depo-Provera may be very suitable for women with an irregular lifestyle for whom contraception is very important – but condoms should also be used (5).

B8   1 – T
    2 – T
    3 – T
    4 – T
    5 – F

A body mass index (BMI) of 40 or over is the definition of "morbid obesity" and has well-known cardiovascular and metabolic complications. A BMI of over 30 is a risk factor for venous thromboembolism (1).

B9 1 – T
2 – F
3 – T
4 – T
5 – F

With the reduced fertility in this age group the coil remains effective for longer than in younger women. These women should be appropriately counselled (1).

If a woman over 40 years of age has no risk factors (e.g. family history, smoking) for cardiovascular disease, she may be allowed to continue either the combined oral contraceptive or the progesterone-only pill if that is her choice (2).

It is the oestrogen that is implicated in the aetiology of thrombotic episodes (3).

There is a possibility of occasional ovulation during the year after the last period (4).

Depot medroxyprogesterone acetate (DMPA) has an adverse effect on high-density lipoprotein-C (HDL-C). It could also possibly be a factor in bone density loss related to hypo-oestrogenism. Irregular bleeding in this age group would require investigation, and the onset of the menopause could be masked (5).

B10 1 – F
2 – F
3 – T
4 – T
5 – T

The Yuzpe regimen can be doubled in dose to ensure adequate steroid plasma levels. Nausea and/or vomiting more than 3 hours after the dose suggests that these levels have been reached (1).

Depot medroxyprogesterone acetate (DMPA) can be prescribed every 8 weeks to ensure adequate contraceptive efficacy (2).

This method suppresses ovulation and should control premenstrual exacerbation of any medical condition (3).

When hepatic-enzyme-inducing drugs are discontinued it can take some weeks for the liver's excretory function to return to normal (5).

Reference: Guillebaud J (1991). Practical prescribing of the combined oral contraceptive pill. In: Filshie M, Guillebaud J (eds) *Contraception – Science and Practice*. Butterworths, London.

B11 1 – F
    2 – F
    3 – F
    4 – T
    5 – T

Condoms are moderately popular with Hindus. Intrauterine devices (IUDs) are preferred in spite of taboos about menstruation (1).

Islam does allow termination of pregnancy in circumstances such as risk to the life to the mother (2).

Sikhism allows sterilisation but the method is not popular (3).

B12 1 – F
    2 – T
    3 – F
    4 – F
    5 – F

See the document on confidentiality and people under 16, issued jointly by the British Medical Association, General Medical Services Committee, Health Education Authority, Brook Advisory Centre, Family Planning Association and the Royal College of General Practitioners.

B13 1 – T
    2 – F
    3 – T
    4 – F
    5 – F

Oral progestogens are useful only in anovulatory dysfunctional uterine bleeding (2).

The most common cause of menorrhagia is idiopathic, not hormonal imbalance (4).

Female sterilisation does not lead to menorrhagia unless the woman had been on the pill and stopped it after sterilisation, in which case the periods may get heavier (5).

B14 1 – T
    2 – F
    3 – T
    4 – F
    5 – T

Ovarian follicular activity commences if the combined oral contraceptive (COC) is omitted for more than 7 days (1).

The CSM guidelines of October 1995 recommended that women with severe varicose veins should not be prescribed gestodene or desogestrel COCs (2).

The risk of arterial disease becomes significantly higher in smokers over the age of 35, with a 21-fold increase in risk compared with non-smokers (3).

Migraine with focal symptoms may indicate transient cerebral ischaemia, therefore oestrogen-containing contraceptive pills, which might precipitate a thrombic stroke, are absolutely contra-indicated (4).

Reference: Clinical and Scientific Committee of the Faculty of Family Planning (1995). *Statement on combined oral contraceptive pills and venous thromboembolism.* Dec. (5).

B15 1 – F
2 – T
3 – T
4 – F
5 – F

The Leiden mutation of coagulation factor V occurs in 20–40% of patients with recurrent venous thrombosis (1).

It causes activated protein C resistance (4).

A definite history of venous thromboembolism in a sibling or parent below the age of 50, or arterial disease below 35 years, warrants screening procedures in patients intending to start using combined oral contraceptives (COCs) (5).

Reference: Machin SJ *et al.* (1995). *British Journal of Family Planning* **21**, 13–14.

B16 1 – T
2 – T
3 – F
4 – T
5 – F

There is no evidence that the combined pill (COC) has a direct effect on cervical intraepithelial neoplasia (CIN) (3).

The COC provides some protection against benign breast lesions (5).

B17 1 – T
2 – F
3 – T
4 – F
5 – T

The combined pill reduces pelvic inflammatory disease by 50% (1).
It has no effect on eczematous skin conditions (2).
The most important non-contraceptive benefit is a 50% reduction in ovarian cancer (3).
Although the Royal College of General Practitioners' study shows a reduction in peptic ulceration, the association is not well-established (4).
The reduction in benign breast disease is substantial, but may be more apparent with progestogen-dominant pills (5).

B18 1 – T
2 – F
3 – T
4 – F
5 – T

Combined pills (COCs) containing gestodene or desogestrel are useful in treating acne, but under the new Committee on Safety of Medicines' guidelines (October 1995), should not be used as first-line contraception. The Faculty of Family Planning subsequently stated that women who have had beneficial effects from such COCs may continue them as long as they are aware of the increased risk of venous thrombosis (October, 1995). Levonorgestrel-containing COCs carry a lower risk (15 per 100 000 women) of venous thromboembolism than COCs containing gestodene or desogestrel (30 per 100 000 women).
Reference: Jick *et al.* (1995). *Lancet* **346**, 1589–1593.
Third-generation progestogens have very minor effects on insulin secretion (2).
The 10-fold differences may account for failures when a pill is missed (3).
Only if diabetic complications are present is the COC absolutely contraindicated (4).
Ascorbic acid at doses of 0.5–1 g/day compete with ethinyloestradiol at the bowel wall for conjugation to sulphate so that more of the steroid is absorbed (5).

B19 1 – T
2 – T
3 – T
4 – F
5 – F

The progesterogen-only pill (POP) contains lower levels of progestogen than the combined oral contraceptive (COC) (1).

Antibiotics have no effect on blood levels of progestogens (2).

Data from the Oxford FPA study showed that women aged 25–29 years have a failure rate of 3.1 per 100 women years. Women aged 40 or over have a failure rate of 0.3 per 100 women years (3).

Femulen contains ethynodiol diacetate (4).

At present, like the COC pill, the POP cannot be prescribed after a hydatidiform mole until the urine is free from human chorionic gonadotrophin (hCG) (5).

B20 1 – T
2 – T
3 – T
4 – F
5 – T

One of the main methods of action of progesterogen-only pills (POPs) is thickening of the cervical mucus, making it impenetrable by sperm. This effect occurs very quickly, and also wears off very quickly. However, it is important to remember that the missed pill guidelines advise 7 days' extra precautions after a missed POP, to keep advice in line with that for COCs. Discretion must be used when deciding which advice is right for which patient (1).

There are probably several reasons for menstrual disturbance. One may be extremely thin, atrophic endometrium; another may be fluctuating hormone levels produced by the functional ovarian cysts. These cysts are common and often asymptomatic, but their presence may be confirmed by ultrasonography (2, 3).

POPs are an excellent contraceptive during lactation as long as the mother is a consistent pill taker (4).

There is definite improvement in flushes on 5 mg/day norethisterone. Evidence that there is enough progestogen in POP to have the same effect is anecdotal (5).

Reference: Paterson M *et al.* (1982). *Br J Obstet Gynaecol* **89**, 464–472.

B21 1 – T
2 – T
3 – F
4 – F
5 – T

The progestogen-only pill (POP) is ideal for diabetics (2).

The POP does not appear to reduce the volume of milk in lactation. Studies on the blood of breast-fed infants have been unable to demonstrate any progestogen levels (3).

No significant effects on clotting have been demonstrated, therefore the POP does not need to be stopped before surgery (4).

As the POP alters the cervical mucus there is some protection against PID (5).

B22 1 – T
2 – F
3 – F
4 – F
5 – T

An intrauterine device (IUD) can be fitted up to 5 days from the earliest calculated date of ovulation (1).

The prevalence of vomiting is around 20% (2).

There is no difference in medical safety between an IUD and emergency hormonal contraception for diabetic women (3).

A combined pill can be started on the first day of the following period (4).

B23 1 – F
2 – T
3 – T
4 – F
5 – F

Postcoital contraception (PCC) is not indicated if up to three tablets are missed mid-cycle as long as at least seven tablets have been taken correctly before this. Ovarian activity will have been inhibited short term (1).

Broad-spectrum antibiotics may interfere with the absorption of oestrogens and therefore the postcoital dose should be increased (2).

Ovulation may be postponed by the previous postcoital treatment. Therefore PCC may be needed again. An intrauterine device could also be considered (3).

A very small teratogenic risk to the fetus cannot be ruled out, but the UK National Association of Family Planning Doctors' series of 50 full-term pregnancies following hormonal PCC showed only one abnormality, which may not have been related. Also, if the Yuzpe method is used, the hormones will not reach the blastocyst as it will not yet have been implanted in the endometrium (4).

The effect on the cervical mucus is at its maximum about 4 hours after taking the POP and gradually diminishes. At 24 hours some sperm penetrability has returned (5).

B24 1 – F
    2 – F
    3 – T
    4 – T
    5 – T

The injectable contraceptives depot medroxyprogesterone acetate (DMPA) and norethisterone enanthate (NET-EN), have three main modes of action. These progestogens inhibit ovulation by action predominantly at the hypothalamic level. This makes the method suitable for women with a past history of ectopic pregnancies (1).

Ovulation inhibition suppresses the formation of functional ovarian cysts, but some degree of endogenous oestradiol production continues (2).

Injectable contraceptives suppress the endometrium, thereby preventing implantation (4).

They thicken the cervical mucus, thereby reducing the incidence of pelvic inflammatory disease (but not sexually transmitted diseases) (5).

B25 1 – T
    2 – F
    3 – T
    4 – F
    5 – F

The injectable contraceptives exhibit first-order kinetics; that is, initial high plasma levels followed by exponential decay (1).

Depot medroxyprogesterone acetate (DMPA) is a derivative of 17-α-hydroxyprogesterone in an aqueous microcrystalline suspension (2). The microcrystals remain at the injection site and are gradually eroded at the surface to release the active steroid (2, 3).

Excessive massaging at the injection site may cause rapid early absorption and metabolism (5).

B26 1 – F
    2 – F
    3 – F
    4 – F
    5 – F

Progestogen-only contraceptives, including depot medroxyprogesterone acetate (DMPA), have very few absolute contraindications. Severe obesity is a relative contraindication, as weight gain is a known side-effect of these contraceptives (1).

DMPA does not compromise lactation (2).

Hepatic-enzyme-inducing drugs (including phenytoin) increase the metabolism of DMPA, which should be given every 8 weeks to ensure adequate contraception (3).

DMPA does not adversely affect liver function, nor does it influence coagulation or fibrinolysis and therefore it can be used in patients with a higher risk of arterial thrombosis, as in sytemic lupus erythematosus (SLE) (4, 5).

B27 1 – F
    2 – F
    3 – T
    4 – T
    5 – F

The contraceptive dose of depot medroxyprogesterone acetate (DMPA) is 150 mg intramuscularly every 12 weeks (1).

In 1995 the licensing arrangements were broadened, making DMPA a first-choice method of contraception (2).

Enuresis may recur secondary to the relaxing effect of progestogens on smooth muscle (4).

Past concerns derived from a study which demonstrated that two out of 12 rhesus monkeys given 50 times the human dose in a 10-year trial developed endometrial cancer. However, high doses of DMPA have been used in the treatment of endometrial cancer (5).

B28 1 – T
    2 – T
    3 – F
    4 – T
    5 – T

Because over 50% of users will become amenorrhoeic by the end of the first year, the method is very useful for women with dysfunctional uterine bleeding (2).

There is no correlation between bleeding irregularities on the progestogen-only pill and with depot medroxyprogesterone acetate (DMPA) (3).

Initial bleeding irregularities can be treated with the combined oral contraceptive pill, "natural" oestrogens and earlier repeat injections of DMPA. There is no good evidence that these methods will improve bleeding patterns in the long term. Pretreatment counselling is therefore of paramount importance (4).

Menstrual irregularity and unpredictable (or no) ovulation may persist for many months after the last injection. There is no evidence that DMPA causes persistent amenorrhoea or permanent infertility (5).

B29 1 – F
    2 – F
    3 – F
    4 – F
    5 – T

Contraceptive vaginal rings have been produced containing levonorgestrel, natural progesterone and combined desogestrel with ethinyl-oestradiol (1).

The levonorgestrel ring is worn continuously for 90 days, and releases 20 µg levonorgestrel/day. It is allowable to remove it during intercourse. The WHO have been studying a natural-progesterone-releasing ring, specifically for use by lactating mothers. It releases 5–10 mg/day of progesterone and lasts for 3 months. The combined desogestrel–ethinyl-oestradiol ring is worn for 3 weeks and removed for the fourth week to allow for a withdrawal bleed. Alternatively, it can be used tricyclically, removing it for a week after 9 weeks' continuous use (2).

The unexpected side-effect has been the appearance of asymptomatic erythematous patches on the vaginal wall. As the cause of these patches is unknown, they have delayed the general availability of the method while further studies are undertaken (3).

The rings do not need to fit over the cervix specifically as in the case of the diaphragm. The ring moves freely within the vagina, and absorption of the active hormone is through any part of the vaginal mucosa. The ring is 5–6 cm in diameter (4).

B30 1 – F
2 – F
3 – F
4 – T
5 – F

Anenorrhoea occurs in 10% of women in the first year of use (1).

Progestogen levels remain constant on a daily basis, which ensures excellent contraceptive efficacy (2).

Follicular development occurs in most cycles, although ovulation may be suppressed (3).

B31 1 – F
2 – T
3 – T
4 – F
5 – T

The implant consists of six capsules (1).

Up to 80% of women will experience menstrual disturbance during the first year of use (2).

Norplant is an expensive form of contraception at the time of fitting, but breaks even compared with a third-generation combined oral contraceptive or depot medroxyprogesterone acetate at 3.5 years of use (4).

Easy removal depends on good insertion, but is likely to take longer than insertion; this should be discussed during preinsertion counselling (5).

B32 1 – T
2 – F
3 – F
4 – T
5 – T

Norplant may improve endometriosis as it can suppress endometrial proliferation (1).

Each rod contains 38 mg of levonorgestrel. The implants release 40 μg/day after the first few weeks, falling to 30 μg/day at 5 years (2).

There is a very low ectopic pregnancy rate (0.08/100 women per year) even if there has been a previous ectopic pregnancy (3).

It suppresses ovulation in approximately 50% of menstrual cycles. If ovulation does occur the luteal phase is often deficient and fertilisation is inhibited (4).

Mood change may occur in 5–10% of women – possibly depression. Removal of Norplant relieves this unwanted effect rapidly (5).

B33 1 – F
2 – T
3 – F
4 – T
5 – T

The risk of infection with intrauterine devices (IUDs) rises in the 20 days following insertion, but drops beyond that (1).

The consensus view is that *Actinomyces*-like organisms on cervical smears indicate replacement or removal of the IUD, though some experts do not agree with this recommendation (2).

If an IUD is removed in mid-cycle, there is a risk of pregnancy unless the woman abstains or uses an alternative method of contraception for the 7 days before removal (3).

B34 1 – F
2 – F
3 – F
4 – F
5 – T

Intrauterine devices (IUDs) in general can be replaced at any time (1).

IUDs do not cause ectopic pregnancy; they actually reduce the risk of ectopics compared with the non-contracepted population. However, more of the IUD failures tend to be ectopic pregnancies (2).

Sampling the endometrium using an endometrial sampler such as a Pipelle does not interfere with the position of an IUD (3).

The perforation risk with IUDs is 1 in 1000 (4).

The third-generation copper IUDs, containing around 380 mm copper, have a lower failure risk (5).

B35 1 – T
2 – F
3 – T
4 – T
5 – F

Removal of the copper intrauterine device (IUD) in early pregnancy reduces the spontaneous abortion rate from 54 to 20% – thus reducing the risk of second trimester abortions, which have a higher risk of complications such as infection and haemorrhage (1).

Nulliparous women have a higher expulsion rate for all types of IUD (2).

All types of IUD cause an increase of leucocytes in the endometrial, uterine and tubular fluids. There is a foreign body reaction involving an increase in all the expected types of white cell (3).

An IUD may be used in a woman who has had a subacute bacterial endocarditis without an anatomical heart lesion or prosthetic heart valve. Antibiotic cover should be used (4).

IUDs are preferably inserted from the last 2–3 days of menstruation until mid-cycle – or up to 5 days after calculated ovulation as a postcoital insertion (5).

B36 1 – T
2 – T
3 – F
4 – T
5 – F

An IUD provides immediate contraception (3).

B37 1 – T
2 – T
3 – T
4 – F
5 – T

Studies have shown that pre-ejaculate can contain sperm although in small numbers (1).

Following ovulation, the ovum survives for 12–24 hours (4).

B38 1 – F
    2 – T
    3 – T
    4 – F
    5 – T

The cervix moves upwards in the pelvis during the fertile phase and is highest at peak oestrogen levels (1).

Using both temperature changes and changes in cervix and mucus is a reliable method (3).

Basal body temperature is raised by 0.2–0.6°C in response to increased progesterone produced by the corpus luteum after ovulation. It therefore marks the end of the fertile phase (4).

Reference: The European Natural Family Planning Study Group (1993). Prospective European multi-centre study of natural family planning (1989–92): interim results. *Adv Contracept* **9**, 269–283.

B39 1 – T
    2 – T
    3 – F
    4 – F
    5 – T

In Japan 50% of married couples use condoms (1).

Double Dutch is being promoted particularly to teenagers to protect against sexually transmitted diseases (2).

Oil-based lubricants such as baby oil will reduce tensile strength (3).

Nystatin gel will, but not the pessaries (4).

Like caps and diaphragms, condoms will reduce the risk of cervical dyskaryosis in women (5).

B40 1 – T
    2 – F
    3 – F
    4 – T
    5 – T

The Femidom does not rely on penile erection for correct use, and can therefore be introduced at any time before intercourse (2).

It is lubricated with dimethicone, which is a silicone-based lubricant (3).

References: Voeller B *et al.* (1991). Gas, dye and viral transport through polyurethane condoms. Letter to the Editor. *JAMA* **226**, 21; Drew WL *et al.* (1990). Evaluation of the virus permeability in a new condom for women. *Sexually Transmitted Diseases* **17**, 110–112 (4).

It is the latex rubber used to manufacture male condoms and diaphragms that is damaged by oil-based lubricants, not the polyurethane used in Femidom (5).

B41 1 – T
    2 – T
    3 – T
    4 – F
    5 – T

Cervical caps are thimble shaped and stay in place by suction so correct size is important. There are four sizes: 22 mm, 25 mm, 28 mm and 31 mm (1).

In the Oxford FPA study, the rate per 1000 woman-years for oral contraceptive users for cervical dyskaryosis was 0.95 and for the diaphragm cap 0.23 (2).

Caps and diaphragms should be left in for 6 hours after intercourse (4).

The Vimule has a high narrow dome and a wide flat side and so is more appropriate for a longer cervix (5).

B42 1 – F
    2 – T
    3 – T
    4 – F
    5 – T

Diaphragms are associated with increased urinary tract infections – probably related to pressure. Changing to a cervical cap is advised (1).

The use of the cap may alter the vaginal flora (3).

Caps and diaphragms do not give protection against human immunodeficiency virus and other sexually transmitted viruses or diseases like syphilis, which may infect the vulva (4).

Extra spermicide is advised if intercourse takes place more than 3 hours after cap insertion (5).

B43 1 – T
    2 – F
    3 – T
    4 – F
    5 – T

Although spermicides can be absorbed through the vaginal wall, recent studies have not shown any teratogenicity (1, 2).

Foaming tablets need to be inserted 10 minutes before intercourse to allow sufficient foam to build up (4).

In a study by Zipper *et al.*, 80 mg propranolol tablets gave a failure rate of only 3.9 per 100 woman-years.

Reference: Zipper J *et al.* (1983). *BMJ* **287**, 1245 (5).

B44 1 – F
    2 – T
    3 – F
    4 – F
    5 – F

Counselling is an important part of vasectomy care at any age, but there is no lower age limit, as long as all the consequences and alternatives have been considered (1).

In sterilisation of either partner only the individual undergoing the operation is required to consent to the procedure (3).

There was a fear that men who had had a vasectomy were more prone to genital cancer. Recent research has shown this to be untrue for testicular cancer, but the causal relation between vasectomy and prostate cancer was inconclusive.

Reference: Møller H *et al.* (1994). *BMJ* **309**, 295–298 (4).

There is no effect on libido in either direction following vasectomy (5).

B45 1 – T
    2 – T
    3 – F
    4 – F
    5 – F

The failure rate includes 1–2 intrauterine pregnancies and 1 ectopic pregnancy per 1000 operations (2).

Pregnancy results in increased vascularity and thickening of the fallopian tubes. Hence there is an increased risk of intra-abdominal bleeding. If the procedure is performed, two clips should be applied to each tube (3).

An intrauterine device should not be removed until at least 7 days after the last act of sexual intercourse. Sperm can survive up to 6 days (4).

The procedure involves only the application of a clip to the fallopian tube. A portion of each fallopian tube is excised during a Pomeroy procedure (5).

B46 1 – T
2 – F
3 – F
4 – T
5 – F

The prostaglandin has to be administered 2 days after the RU-486. A complete abortion occurs in over 95% of women (2).

The dose recommended by the manufacturers to achieve abortion is 600 mg (3).

Reference: Webb A. *et al.* (1992). *BMJ* **305**, 927–931 (4).

Mifepristone used alone will induce abortion in 3% of women (5).

B47 1 – F
2 – F
3 – T
4 – F
5 – T

The Human Fertilisation and Embryology Bill amended the 1967 Abortion Act by restricting abortion to 24 weeks if "the continuation of the pregnancy would involve risk, greater than if the pregnancy were terminated, of injury to the physical or mental health of the pregnant woman/any existing child(ren) of the family of the pregnant woman" (clauses C and D). However, when there is serious risk to the mother's life or a substantial chance of serious handicap (clauses A, B and D) there is no upper limit. See form HSA1 (revised 1991) (1).

Two doctors' signatures are always required for a legal abortion (2).

There is no association between first trimester surgical abortion and cervical incompetence (4).

B48 1 – F
2 – F
3 – T
4 – F
5 – T

Cervical cytology is not essential when assessing a woman presenting with an unplanned pregnancy (1).
The risk of postabortion infection is around 3–5% (2).
The risk of serious complication, such as perforation or severe pelvic inflammatory disease, is around 1% (4).

B49 1 – F
2 – T
3 – F
4 – T
5 – F

There are many types of loss, physical and otherwise. The wrong dosage of pill can have physical complications; giving the pill when there are contraindications can cause, for example, stroke; failing to give proper instruction of, for example, caps can lead to misuse and consequent pregnancies which is a loss in itself for which damages can be claimed (1).

This is an accurate précis of the Scottish decision in *Hunter* v. *Hamley* and the English decision of *Bolam* v. *Frien Hospital Management Committee* (2).

It is no defence that the doctor acted in good faith for the best interests of the patient. Patients are entitled to choose their own medical treatment and are entitled to choose options which the doctor thinks is not best for the patient. Sterilisation without consent is an assault (3).

Consent to all forms of medical treatment is legally valid only if it is personal consent. The only exception to this is that parents can consent on behalf of children who do not themselves have the capacity to consent (NB: the law of Scotland is very different from the law of England on children's capacity to consent) (4).

In Scotland abortion can only be performed (legally speaking) upon a pregnant woman, and until the fertilised egg has implanted there is no pregnant women: so any action before implantation cannot be abortion. In England the matter is a little more complicated because criminal abortion ("attempting to induce a miscarriage") can be committed even when there is no pregnancy (because the attempt can still be made). However, the prosecution authorities take the view that postcoital contraception is not abortion and will never be charged as such (5).

Section C – Reproductive Health Care

1. BREAST

C1 Concerning the breast:

1. every woman on hormonal treatment of any kind should have an annual breast examination by a doctor or a nurse
2. every woman should have mammography before starting hormone replacement therapy (HRT)
3. during breast examination, visual inspection is as important as manual palpation
4. women developing breast cancer under the age of 45 have a 50% chance of having a genetic abnormality of the long arm of chromosome 17
5. recent research suggesting that patients with breast cancer operated on in the first half of the menstrual cycle have a worse prognosis than those operated on in the last half of the cycle has been validated by subsequent research

C2 With regard to mastalgia:

1. cyclical mastalgia is more difficult to treat than non-cyclical mastalgia
2. in the treatment of cyclical mastalgia, evening primrose oil has been shown to be significantly superior to placebo in double-blind studies
3. danazol is less effective than oil of evening primrose in the treatment of cyclical mastalgia
4. a postmenopausal woman with non-cyclical mastalgia should be referred to a breast clinic
5. cyclical mastalgia is a known side-effect of hormone replacement therapy

2. COLPOSCOPY

C3   Abnormalities of the cervix seen at colposcopy:

1. include aceto-white-positive areas on the transformation zone
2. include iodine-positive areas on the transformation zone
3. include punctation
4. are best examined through a green filter if vascular
5. allow a diagnosis of cervical intraepithelial neoplasia (CIN) to be made

C4   The normal postmenopausal cervix may:

1. exhibit contact bleeding
2. have pearly aceto-white patches
3. show poor uptake of iodine
4. be polypoid
5. be better assessed after a course of oestrogen

C5   The following are colposcopic features of high-grade cervical neoplasia:

1. double capillaries
2. "leopard" spots appearance after Schiller's iodine application
3. fused columnar villi
4. coarse punctation
5. visible gland openings

3. GENITOURINARY MEDICINE

C6   Bacterial vaginosis:

1. often yields *Gardnerella vaginalis*
2. is associated with an increase in vaginal pH
3. lactobacilli are present in large numbers on a Gram-stained vaginal smear from a patient with it
4. oral metronidazole is an effective treatment for it
5. it is considered mandatory to treat the male sexual partner of a female with it

C7 Chlamydia:

1. *Chlamydia trachomatis* is an obligate intracellular parasite
2. *Chlamydia trachomatis* is to be considered a pathogen at all times
3. *Chlamydia trachomatis* is a common cause of infertility
4. *Chlamydia* serology is a helpful diagnostic test
5. the β-lactams are first-line antibiotics for the treatment of chlamydial infections

C8 Genital herpes:

1. results exclusively from herpes simplex type 2 (HSV2) infection
2. may present as retention of urine
3. may be confused with candidal vulvitis which should be considered in the differential diagnosis
4. lesions are non-infectious once crusts form
5. attack can be aborted by acyclovir prophylaxis

C9 Genital warts:

1. positive serology is the gold standard for diagnosis of exposure
2. genital warts are a marker for the presence of other sexually transmitted diseases
3. the progressive potential of minor cervical atypia is influenced by human papilloma virus (HPV) type
4. cervical warts indicate colposcopy referral
5. infective genital wart virus is found only in the superficial differentiated layers of the epithelium

C10 Gonorrhoea:

1. *Neisseria gonorrhoeae* is a Gram-positive organism
2. gonococcal genital tract infection in women is often asymptomatic
3. a high vaginal swab is the appropriate specimen for microbiological tests
4. systemic gonococcal infection is rare
5. is always sensitive to penicillin

C11 Human immunodeficiency virus (HIV) infection:

1. active infection with other sexually transmitted bacterial and viral diseases increases the risk of acquiring HIV
2. active infection with other sexually transmitted bacterial and viral diseases increases the risk of transmitting HIV
3. the major spread of HIV is homosexual
4. sexual transmission is easier via anal than vaginal intercourse
5. the risk of transmission from woman to man is higher than from man to woman

C12 Syphilis:

1. the causative organism is *Treponema pertenue*
2. a simple, painless, indurated genital ulcer should be considered syphilitic until proven otherwise
3. the causative organism can be cultured on blood agar
4. condylomata acuminata are pathognomonic of secondary syphilis
5. penicillin resistance is not an issue when treating patients with syphilis

C13 Vaginal discharge:

1. *Trichomonas vaginalis* is a sexually transmitted infection
2. *Trichomonas vaginalis* infection is best treated with 4-quinolones
3. vaginal candidiasis is associated with glycosuria
4. *Escherichia coli* is associated with irritating vaginal discharge
5. broad-spectrum antibiotics may exacerbate vaginal candidal infection

4. MENOPAUSE

C14 The following are *absolute* contraindications to the prescription of hormone replacement therapy:

1. a history of deep vein thrombosis
2. untreated breast cancer
3. hypertension
4. heavy smoking
5. a history of myocardial infarction

C15 In the prevention of osteoporosis:

1. the bone-sparing dose of oral oestradiol is 2 mg
2. calcium and vitamin D are especially indicated for white vegetarians
3. progestogens have an antiresorptive activity similar to, but lower than, that of oestrogens
4. a bone mineral density (BMD) of 1 standard deviation below the mean doubles the risk of fracture
5. the lifetime risk of fracture for a 50-year-old woman is 10%

C16 A non-hysterectomised woman taking hormone replacement therapy (HRT):

1. should take a progestogen for 12 days each cycle
2. should not take HRT if her smear shows dyskaryosis
3. should have a plasma oestradiol level of 200–800 pmol/l
4. will probably require a higher dose of oestrogen for cardioprotection than to protect against bone loss
5. should have an endometrial biopsy every 18 months

C17 In the following conditions, transdermal hormone replacement therapy (HRT) is preferable to oral HRT if:

1. there is heavy withdrawal bleeding on oral HRT
2. there is hypertriglyceridaemia
3. the woman is taking phenytoin
4. the woman is taking angiotensin-converting enzyme inhibitors
5. the woman prefers a more natural therapy

5. PREGNANCY

C18 With regard to ectopic pregnancy:

1. the ectopic pregnancy rate is higher in users of intrauterine devices
2. symptoms can include syncopy
3. ectopic pregnancy is the commonest cause of maternal death
4. sterilization is not a factor
5. intratubal methotrexate has been used in the treatment of ectopic pregnancies

C19 Septic abortion:

1. in most cases the infection is localised to the decidua
2. the common causative agent is *Chlamydia trachomatis*
3. the uterus must be evacuated once the pyrexia settles
4. septic shock is a consequence in 5% of cases
5. laparoscopy is indicated to exclude tubal damage

C20 Recurrent miscarriage:

1. affects 5% of fertile women
2. is more likely to be caused by fetal chromosomal abnormalities than sporadic miscarriage
3. bacterial vaginosis is a common cause of early pregnancy loss
4. association with antiphospholipid syndrome has been established
5. suppression of leuteinising hormone secretion may reduce the risk

6. PREMENSTRUAL SYNDROME

C21 In women with premenstrual syndrome:

1. the diagnosis is confirmed by low progesterone levels on day 21
2. luteinising hormone releasing hormone agonists are useful in the diagnosis of severe premenstrual syndrome
3. epilepsy can be exacerbated premenstrually
4. placebo-controlled trials have shown that depot medroxyprogesterone acetate is an effective treatment for premenstrual syndrome
5. the combined contraceptive pill can improve, worsen or have no effect on premenstrual symptoms

7. SEXUAL PROBLEMS

C22 Concerning the normal sexual response:

1. moistening of the vagina during sexual arousal comes from secretions from the Bartholin's glands
2. female orgasm consists of rhythmic contractions of the muscles, occurring at 0.8 second intervals
3. during the plateau phase, the testes shrink and are pulled higher into the scrotum
4. the circumcised man has less control over ejaculation than the uncircumcised man
5. a larger flaccid penis becomes proportionally larger on erection than a smaller flaccid penis

C23 In a psychosexual problem consultation:

1. the effect the patient has on the doctor is irrelevant
2. it is necessary to take a detailed history
3. the "patient" is the couple
4. it is always necessary to examine the patient
5. understanding and resolution of the problem may occur in a single consultation

Answers to Section C

C1 1 – F
    2 – F
    3 – T
    4 – F
    5 – F

Examination either by a doctor or nurse or by the woman herself is notoriously unreliable. The modern trend is to encourage breast awareness; that is, the woman herself becoming very familiar with her own breasts, including how they feel to palpation, and how they change with her menstrual cycle. She should report *any* change from normal (i.e. not just lumps) to her medical advisor. This may not be a very efficient screening method, but it is much better than an annual medical check (1).

Many women begin hormone replacement therapy before the menopause. Mammography is not at all helpful in screening the premenopausal breast, as the tissue is too dense to allow accurate assessment (2).

Visual inspection is far more likely to pick up skin dimpling or skin tethering that manual examination (3).

Between 1 and 6% of women developing breast cancer have a genetic abnormality on chromosome 17. This rises to 4–20% if the cancer develops under the age of 45 (4).

Several centres have repeated the Guy's study of performing the operation for breast cancer in the second half of the menstual cycle, and the results have been conflicting. Some centres found no effect at all; others found a significant result in the opposite direction (5).

C2 1 – F
    2 – T
    3 – F
    4 – T
    5 – T

Cyclical mastalgia will usually respond to a variety of therapies. Evening primrose oil (EPO) should be the first-line therapy and can be prescribed with hormonal contraception. Low-dose danazol is superior to EPO, but has unacceptable side-effects for some women, including androgenic and antioestrogenic effects (2, 3).

Non-cyclical mastalgia is notoriously difficult to treat; however, in post-menopausal women, it can be a sign of underlying breast pathology (4).

Cyclical mastalgia commonly occurs with the combined contraceptive pill and hormone replacement therapy (5).

C3   1 – T
     2 – F
     3 – T
     4 – T
     5 – F

Aceto-white epithelium (aceto-white-positive area) is present when there is increased nuclear activity within the epithelium. This can occur in a physiological state with very immature metaplasia, but is more usually seen associated with cervical intraepithelial neoplasia (CIN) (1).

Epithelium composed of normal squamous cells containing glycogen will take up iodine and therefore give iodine-positive areas. Cells *not* taking up iodine, i.e. not containing glycogen, are likely to be found in the presence of CIN (2).

Increased vascularisation is characteristic of all new growths, both benign and malignant. In CIN the patterns are described as punctation and mosaicism. In punctation, vessels are seen end-on, and look like red full stops against a white background. In mosaicism, the new vessels branch on the surface and form mosaic patterns (3, 4).

Changes seen at colposcopy may indicate whether a lesion is major or minor in severity, but final diagnosis of CIN can be made only by histo-pathology. The colposcope is an aid to diagnosis, but not a diagnostic tool in itself (5).

C4   1 – T
     2 – F
     3 – T
     4 – F
     5 – T

The postmenopausal cervix suffers from thinning of the epithelium and therefore bleeds easily (1).

It is neither polypoid nor pearly white (2, 4).

It also has poor glycogen content and therefore has a poor uptake of iodine (3).

Local or systemic oestrogens allow better quality smears and a more satisfactory colposcopy (5).

C5 1 – F
2 – F
3 – F
4 – T
5 – F

Double capillaries are a normal feature of cervical tissue sometimes seen in cervicitis (1).

The "leopard" spots appearance of the cervix is associated with trichomoniasis (2).

Fusion of columnar villi is a normal feature of squamous metaplasia, as are visible gland openings (3, 5).

C6 1 – T
2 – T
3 – F
4 – T
5 – F

Anaerobes and *Gardnerella* are the usual organisms found on bacterial cultures, but *Gardnerella* is a commensal in 20% of women (1).

Vaginal pH is often alkaline in bacterial vaginosis – a reflection of abnormal microflora (reduced lactobacilli) (2).

The presence of large numbers of lactobacilli on a Gram-stained smear is an index of a healthy vagina (3).

Metronidazole is the treatment of choice for bacterial vaginosis (4).

There is no evidence that seeing or offering treatment to the male partner has any place in the management (5).

C7 1 – T
2 – T
3 – T
4 – F
5 – F

Chlamydia can only survive using the columnar epithelial cells' own mechanisms – metabolic, enzymic (1).

Chlamydia should never be considered to be a commensal (2).

Reference: Westrom L (1994). Sexually Transmitted Diseases and

Infertility. *Sexually Transmitted Disease 1994*. IRL Press (3).

Chlamydia serology is indicative of *past* infection, i.e. it is a "stable door" test (4).

First-line antibiotics are tetracyclines and the macrolides (5).

C8 1 – F
    2 – T
    3 – T
    4 – T
    5 – T

Herpes simplex virus (HSV) is a double-stranded DNA virus – there are type 1 and type 2. Type 1 usually causes cold sores, etc. – but is increasingly the cause of genital herpes (1).

Urinary retention may be caused by extreme dysuria or occasionally viral infection of the sacral autonomic plexus (2).

Viral shedding stops once crusts form over the lesion (4).

Recurrences can be prevented with continuous use of acyclovir, but the long-term safety data are not yet available (5).

C9 1 – F
    2 – T
    3 – T
    4 – T
    5 – T

Genital warts are sexually transmitted. *Ipso facto*, they are a marker for other sexual infections (2).

Human papilloma virus (HPV) types 16 and 18 are implicated in the progression of cervical atypia (3).

Cervical warts may be associated with cervical intraepithelial neoplasia (CIN), hence colposcopy is appropriate (4).

The virus infects the keratinocyte, which is above the basement membrane (5).

C10 1 – F
     2 – T
     3 – F
     4 – T
     5 – F

Neisseria gonorrhoeae is a Gram-negative diplococcus (1).

The site of infection in women is the endocervix or more rarely the urethra, and ever more rarely the rectum, and gonococcal infection at these sites is "silent" (2).

The gonococcus infects columnar, not stratified, squamous epithelium (3).

Less than 1% of gonococcal infections exhibit systemic manifestations (4).

Some strains of *Neisseria gonorrhoeae* produce penicillinase (5).

C11 1 – T
      2 – T
      3 – F
      4 – T
      5 – F

Worldwide 70% of cases are heterosexually acquired (3).

Anal intercourse is more traumatic than vaginal intercourse (4).

C12 1 – F
      2 – T
      3 – F
      4 – F
      5 – T

The causative organism is *Treponema pallidum* (1).

Painless indurated single genital ulcer is almost certainly a chancre (2).

It has never been proved possible to culture the treponema of infectious syphilis on agar (3).

Condylomata acuminata are genital warts. Condylomata lata are pathognomonic of secondary syphilis (4).

Treponema pallidum has never lost its sensitivity to penicillin (5).

C13 1 – T
      2 – F
      3 – T
      4 – F
      5 – T

Trichomonas infection is treated with metronidazole (2).

Candida is a fungus that thrives on glucose (3).

Broad spectrum antibiotics kill lactobacilli present in a healthy vagina, allowing *Candida* to flourish (5).

C14 1 – F
2 – T
3 – F
4 – F
5 – F

There are very few absolute contraindications to hormone replacement therapy, but active breast cancer is one, and so is undiagnosed abnormal genital tract bleeding. Many things previously considered contraindications, such as cardiovascular risk factors, are now considered positive indications.

C15 1 – T
2 – F
3 – F
4 – T
5 – F

Vitamin D is indicated in risk groups such as Asian women not adequately exposed to the sun (2).

Progestogens have an osteoblast-stimulating effect (3).

The lifetime risk of fracture for a 50-year-old woman is 40% (5).

C16 1 – T
2 – F
3 – T
4 – T
5 – F

The use of cyclical progestogen is protective for the endometrium (1).

Hormone replacement therapy (HRT) does not affect the risk of cervical neoplasia (2).

An endometrial biopsy is not indicated as long as the woman is on a combined oestrogen–progestogen preparation and has regular withdrawal bleeds (5).

C17 1 – F
2 – T
3 – T
4 – T
5 – F

Heavy withdrawal bleeds are uncommon on hormone replacement

therapy (HRT). If they occur the route of administration is of no specific consequence (1).

Oral HRT increases triglyceride levels in the first pass through the liver; therefore, transdermal HRT may have an advantage in patients with hypertriglyceridaemia (2).

The same applies to women taking phenytoin. Theoretically, the use of transdermal preparations is less vulnerable to the effect of liver-enzyme-inducing drugs (3).

Angiotensin-converting enzyme (ACE) inhibitors are used for the treatment of hypertension. They have no interactions with transdermal hormone replacement, but some authorities prefer the use of transdermal oestrogen in a woman with hypertension as there is less likelihood of interference with the renin–angiotensin system (4).

Transdermal HRT is no more natural than oral HRT (5).

C18 1 – T
      2 – T
      3 – F
      4 – F
      5 – T

The ectopic pregnancy rate in the UK is 1 in 200 pregnancies. This increases to 1 in 10 to 1 in 30 pregnancies in users of intrauterine devices (IUDs). However, as the overall pregnancy rate in IUD users is low (0.5 per hundred woman-years or less with the new copper and levonorgestrel IUDs), the risk of an ectopic pregnancy is consequently very low (1).

Symptoms include unilateral abdominal pain, amenorrhoea, abnormal vaginal bleeding and shoulder pain (2).

Ectopic pregnancy is the third commonest cause of maternal death after hypertensive disease of pregnancy and thromboembolism (3).

Sterilisation is a factor in ectopic pregnancy. If one fallopian tube is partially occluded there is a risk that an ovum may be fertilised but unable to progress satisfactorily along the tube (4).

Intratubal methotrexate has been successfully used in the conservative management of ectopic pregnancies. It is not standard practice in the UK (5).

C19 1 – T
      2 – F
      3 – F

4 – T

5 – F

The causative agents of septic abortion are anaerobic Gram-negative bacteria (2).

The uterus is best evacuated early once antibiotic cover is established (3).

There is no indication for laparoscopy in the management of un-complicated septic abortion (5).

C20 1 – F

2 – F

3 – F

4 – T

5 – T

Recurrent miscarriage affects 1% of fertile women (1).

Fetal chromosomal abnormalities are a much more likely cause of sporadic miscarriage than of recurrent miscarriage (2).

Bacterial vaginosis is an important cause of late miscarriage and premature rupture of the membrane (3).

20% of recurrent miscarriages are associated with the antiphospho-lipid syndrome (4).

Luteinising hormone is believed to cause early miscarriage in women with polycystic ovarian disease (5).

C21 1 – F

2 – T

3 – T

4 – F

5 – T

The diagnosis is based on prospective daily recording of symptoms by the patient (1).

Luteinising hormone releasing hormone (LHRH) agonists are very useful in suppressing symptoms, but antioestrogenic side-effects preclude long-term use (2).

The syndrome can be primary or secondary in nature. In secondary premenstrual syndrome (PMS), the symptoms, e.g. epilepsy, asthma and depression, are exacerbated premenstrually (3).

To date there have been no placebo-controlled trials of depot medroxy-progesterone acetate (DMPA). However, anecdotal evidence suggests that it can be useful in primary PMS and in prevention of premenstrual exacerbation of symptoms (4).

The effect of the combined contraceptive pill is unpredictable (5).

C22 1 – F
 2 – T
 3 – F
 4 – F
 5 – F

Lubrication of the vagina occurs by means of a "sweating" reaction through the walls of the vagina (1).

Contractions of the muscles at 0.8 second intervals occur in both men and women during orgasm (2).

During the plateau phase, the testes are pulled higher into the scrotum, but they enlarge, not shrink (3).

During Masters and Johnson's research, circumcised and uncircumcised men were matched at random, and no clinically significant difference was found between the two (4).

Masters and Johnson found that a small penis may double in length on erection, whereas the lengthening of a large penis is less marked (5).

Reference: Masters WH, Johnson VE (1966). *Human Sexual Response.* Little, Brown, Boston.

C23 1 – F
 2 – F
 3 – F
 4 – F
 5 – T

The doctor–patient relationship (the emotions and moods aroused within the consultation) are often central to understanding the problem (1).

A history may or may not be helpful; an unstructured interview following the patient's lead is useful. A study of the "here and now" of the patient's problem is often more revealing than a detailed history (2).

Many patients and doctors hold the belief that to resolve a psychosexual difficulty both partners need to be present. However, experience has shown that the "patient" is the person complaining of the problem; this may even be true if the patient is complaining not about their own sexual life/response, but about their partner's. Working with the doctor–

patient relationship is usually easier in a one-to-one situation (3).

Examination of the patient may be very helpful, leading to a "moment of truth", but sometimes the barriers to examination either being offered or accepted, and a study of why examination was or was not performed, are just as revealing as the actual examination (4).

There is a widely held belief that psychosexual medicine is very time consuming. This is not always the case: the "brief encounter" with speedy resolution of the problem is quite common (5).

Reference: Skrine R (ed.) (1989). *Introduction to Psychosexual Medicine.* Montana Press, Carlisle.